Seven Steps to Heal Your Thyroid

A Proven Plan to Increase Energy, Elevate Mood, and Optimize Weight

By Dr. Meghna Thacker

A Leading Naturopathic Physician, Author, and Inspirational Speaker info@meghnathacker.com

Ordering Information: Quantity sales. Special discounts are available on quantity purchases by corporations, associations, and others. For details, contact the publisher at the email address above.

CONTENTS

STEP - 2
NATUROPATHIC TREATMENTS 27

STEP - 3
HEAL YOUR GUT 53

STEP - 4
REDUCE TOXIC ENVIRONMENTAL EXPOSURE 83

STEP - 5
BALANCE YOUR HORMONES 99

STEP - 6
EMOTIONAL HEALING 129

STEP - 7
THE WHOLE PICTURE 147

DEDICATION

I dedicate this book to you, my reader.

If you are someone who has low energy and has to push yourself to get through your day or suffer from mood swings that may alternate between depression and bursts of anger, or has a difficult time losing weight after trying all the diets and exercise programs out there, then this book is for you.

I have tried to keep this book short and simple to read. I hope that you find the content informative.

I would love to hear from you. There are a few ways to connect with me:

Website: www.meghnathacker.com

Email: info@meghnathacker.com

Facebook Page: *Dr. Meghna Thacker*

THANKS

I thank my husband, Apurva Patel, for his constant love, support, and encouragement. We are blessed with two beautiful boys, Aarav and Kiaan. I thank my parents, Urvashi and Jairaj Thacker, for their unconditional love and courage for letting me leave the comfort of my home in India to live my dream.

I sincerely thank my mentors, Dr. Gino Tutera and Dr. Thomas Kruzel, who not only excelled in their own fields but by example also taught me to be a kind and a compassionate doctor.

Thank you, Parul Agrawal, my book-writing coach, who guided me with the steps I needed to take to write my first book.

Thank you Asif and Harshita Khan from AKreation for the book cover idea and photography and Pro_ebook covers for the book cover design.

Lastly, I thank Jewel Eliese, my developmental editor, who helped me through this entire process, from reviewing my book outline to editing the final draft, Dr. Beth Lynne, who completed the final edits, and Abhishek Tiwari from www.CreativeKindles.com for formatting

TESTIMONIALS

Dr Thacker's book is deeply rooted in the naturopathic philosophy that the body is innately self-healing. "Seven Steps to Heal Your Thyroid" gives the readers a deeper understanding of the root cause and physiology of their symptoms and practical steps to take to begin healing, naturally.

~Razi Berry, Publisher
Naturopathic Doctor News & Review & NaturalPath

Seven Steps to Heal Your Thyroid by Dr. Meghna Thacker is an excellent resource for anyone who no longer is responding to conventional medical therapy for hormone or thyroid problems. Having experienced severe thyroid problems herself, and trained in Naturopathic Medicine to treat the whole person, she is uniquely qualified to address endocrine system imbalances. This book helps one to easily understand this complex subject and empowers them to obtain the help they need. I highly recommend it to anyone wanting to take charge of their health.

~Dr. Thomas A Kruzel, Scottsdale, AZ

Thyroid disease is so prevalent in our society. I see it nearly every day in my practice. In Seven Steps to Heal Your Thyroid, Dr. Thacker outlines easy to follow steps to uncover the issues that may be making you feel sick. By sharing her personal journey, she shows you how to lose weight, gain energy, and repair your health. This book has the answers you need!

~Dr. Ann Lovick , Owner
Valley Natural Medical Center

"Dr. Thacker's "Seven Steps to Heal Your Thyroid" is the best and most comprehensive thyroid book on the market today. The book is easy to understand, informative and a pleasure to read."

~Dr. Shaon Hines

Women have waited too long for the informative, easy to read Seven Steps. We cease to feel unheard, misdiagnosed, and unacknowledged. Seven Steps is a must read that leaves us feeling relieved and empowered.

~Nita Lapinski, Clairvoyant Medium,
Flagstaff, AZ

FOREWORD

It was May of 2006, when I was lecturing at Southwest College of Naturopathic Medicine in Arizona. After the lecture, a young lady with a twinkle in her eyes approached me. She asked me if she could do a preceptorship with me at my clinic in Bellevue, WA. And I said, "Yes, you can preceptor with me." When I came to USA in 1986, I tried to do preceptorships with many MDs and NDs but was refused. At that time, I promised myself if anyone would come to me for a preceptorship, I would never say no. She came to my Bellevue clinic in August of 2006. With her charming personality, she befriended everyone in the clinic. She was adopted into the family and we also invited her to attend a religious ceremony at our home.

Since then, we have also been adopted by her family in Mumbai. We even attended her brother's wedding ceremony in Mumbai, India.

While doing the preceptorship with me at my clinic, Dr. Thacker was very curious and asked lots of questions. Although she had been trained to be a Homeopath in India, she dared to come to USA to learn Naturopathic Medicine. She was trying to grasp Ayurvedic models and thinking parallels to Homeopathy. She was very much intrigued with Ayurvedic medicine and psychosomatic body types. I knew at the time that she would be very successful in her career. She had a keen interest in medicine. I'm not surprised that she is very successful in her practice and now she has embarked in her journey to write a book, Seven Steps to Heal Your Thyroid. This is an excellent guidebook for folks who are suffering with hypothyroidism. She has intricately woven her own life journey and how she healed her Hashimoto's Thyroiditis with a complete understanding of "true natural medicine."

Dr. Thacker starts with her personal story and then talks about the functionality of the thyroid in easy and understandable language. Then she discusses the Naturopathic treatment basics. Treat the cause of the disease. Heal the gut; gut healing has come into the limelight lately with human genome projects. But this is the first step in Ayurvedic medicine. Remove the burden of toxic load from your body, balance the hormones, work on your emotions, and treat the whole person.

I used to have radio show named "Our bodies are our natural pharmacy." Bodies make every known chemical on demand; we are the owners of our bodies' manuals and we shape our realities, including health, disease, happiness, and sorrows. Healing comes from within, and we all are blessed to have healing mechanisms in our bodies. Disease is due to the mistake of intelligence flowing in every cell of our bodies. Dr. Thacker very elegantly explains in easy-to-understand language how to restore the balance and beat hypothyroidism. She is very qualified not only because she has gone to two medical colleges, but she has lived through the disease and healed herself following the same principles that she teaches her patients. Even in my clinic, the most common health issue I face is hypothyroidism. I also got more insights on how to treat thyroid effectively. It is a matter of immense pride and pleasure when your kids or students surpass your expectations and a moment comes when you also learn from them. Dr. Meghna Thacker has done a tremendous job in writing this book in easy-to-understand language, and I am sure readers and patients of hypothyroidism will benefit tremendously. I wish all the best to Dr. Thacker.

With Love,

Virender Sodhi MD (Ayurved) N.D.
Bellevue, WA

MY STORY

I alone cannot change the world, but I can cast a stone across the waters to create many ripples.
~ Mother Teresa

A saint walked into our home. A blue and white sari covered her hair, her face was lined with wrinkles and her eyes were thoughtful. There was something special about this woman. Something that made her little frame seem large, authoritative. Being in her presence made me realize just how she'd started her organization and helped thousands of poor and destitute people around the world with strength and love. Mother Teresa. She became a role model for me. What a great person she was and her work in India was unsurpassed. Her life must have been so hard, but she dedicated it to serving other people, and it is because of her that I have set out to serve others as well, one by one.

I was born in Mumbai, India to a family that dedicated their lives to education and service of the community. They own educational institutions and are very well-respected. Due to the philanthropic work that my grandfather did, it was normal to have public figures like Mother Teresa visit our home. Of course, I went to the school that my family owned and did not always enjoy the special attention by teachers and staff. Mind you, this is a huge school that has 5,000 students. Growing up, my life was that of a Mumbai princess, but sometimes I felt like running away, to just be "Meghna."

My protective and loving family inspired my passions. My mother was ambitious and wanted me to learn Indian classical dance. If I was going to dance, I would do my best like I always strived to do in every area of my life. At the age of 16, I danced a solo three-hour recital. It is called *Arangetram*. I would practice for five hours every single day for a year to get ready for this recital. I learned about life through dance and my Guru, Smt. Kirti Naik. The rigorous training and long performance taught me discipline, perseverance, dedication, and hardwork. I learned about life values and principles through mythological stories depicted through dance. It is part of the reason I had the strength to pursue the rigorous schooling to become a doctor.

For my undergraduate work, I went to homeopathic medical school for five years. I became the president of the Rotaract Club of Homeopathic College and would organize projects like providing dustbins (or trashcans, as Americans call them) for our college campus to promote a clean environment. Trashcans are not easily found in India, so we used this event to raise money and give back to the community by purchasing these dustbins. We also initiated a project with the Missionaries of Charity, which had been started by Mother Teresa. We would raise money and then donate it to the orphanage or collect clothing and give it to the children there. It really broke my heart to see all those little cribs lined up and to think of these children without their parents. It increased my desire to help others.

In my last year of clinical rotations in the homeopathic hospital, I met students from the National College of Naturopathic Medicine that had come to learn homeopathy. I learned about the Naturopathic Medicine program from them. I loved how holistic this program was. I would be able to learn both natural and conventional medicine and upon graduation have a wide toolbox of medicines to choose from. I would be able to individualize the choice of treatment based on every patient, since each patient is unique. I knew right away this was my purpose in life. It was a strong calling. My passion. It was a completion of what I wanted to offer the world and a way to help others. I started dreaming about becoming a Naturopathic Doctor.

I faced many challenges along my journey. I started communicating with all four schools in the US that offered the accredited ND program. All of them helped answer my questions until it came to sponsoring a student visa for me. At that time, none of the schools had had any student applying directly from India. It was the first time for Southwest College of Naturopathic Medicine

(SCNM) as well. I remember Jennifer Brockett, who worked in student enrollment services at that time, was open to understanding the process and helped me step by step to come and study there. Even today, I remember and thank her from my heart.

After coming here, I faced different challenges. Everything was different. I came from this overly protective and well-respected family to a place where I did not know anyone. I rented a studio apartment and completed my six months at the community college before my enrollment at SCNM, while my new husband went to school at Syracuse University in upstate New York. We were apart for three and a half years. My sheltered princess life splintered. I had a lot of growing up to do. I got into challenging relations with friends and learned many life-lessons the hard way. The four-year program was definitely intense, but I enjoyed the hands-on learning. During my clinical rotations, I tried to get as much experience by shadowing doctors from offsite clinics and was interested in finding out what real-world practice would be like.

Besides the coursework being rigorous and demanding, I was also learning how to live all by myself, far away from my family in an entirely new culture. In a way, I was naïve. I had always been taught that everybody is nice, that there's no good and evil. Growing up, I almost never went anywhere alone and was constantly protected. Because of this, I went through a lot of times where I felt like I was taken advantage of because of my kind and big heart. It shattered me emotionally. This happened for many years. It was a challenging time and important learning process, and I believe the stress contributed to my health problems.

I remember feeling exhausted. I struggled to stay awake during the day, yet I couldn't fall asleep at night. Many times, I would end up missing my eight o'clock class, which was very unlike my ambitious personality. I used to put my head down on my desk between classes, and my classmates would ask if something was wrong with me. I would say, "Oh yeah, I'm fine," but internally, I wasn't.

During a visit home to India, my friends and family saw a vast change in me. I'd lost half my hair and had gained weight to the point where I couldn't fit into my jeans anymore. I became depressed and was struggling with life, having to constantly push myself every day just to seem normal. I didn't feel like me anymore, and my friends and family knew something wasn't right. Yet I didn't want to admit to myself that I might have a problem.

After I completed my four-year medical school and graduated as a Naturopathic Physician, I was fortunate to get a preceptorship at Dr. Gino Tutera's clinic. He was an Ob/Gyn. It was also my passion to help women, so working with him and learning his unique way of balancing the hormones really matched what I was looking for in a job and mentor. He was a very kind, compassionate, and knowledgeable doctor with an excellent bedside manner and I was honored to work for him. But between patients, I would get foggy and start shutting down. I then knew I couldn't avoid my symptoms any longer and decided to run comprehensive bloodwork.

My lab values for the thyroid antibodies were off the charts. I was shocked. At first, I thought it had to be a mistake, that these could not be my test results. I was in denial. Dr. Tutera was the one who helped me realize the truth by simply talking with me logically. That was my bloodwork. Those were my results. I finally had to accept it.

I had Hashimoto's Thyroiditis.

After two years of working with Dr. Tutera, I felt like I was missing out on using all the other Naturopathic Modalities. I was scared that I would forget if I did not use them. Then I found Dr. Thomas Kruzel, owner of Rockwood Natural Medicine, and started to build my practice there. It was not easy. To make ends meet, I started working part-time at two other locations. I had taken up a lot of work building my practice out of three different locations. Then I got pregnant with my first child and continued working.

I was diagnosed with Hashimoto's Thyroiditis when I was doing my preceptorship. I was able to control my symptoms of hypothyroidism with natural supplements until after having my first son. Due to my personal struggle with this condition, I researched and learned many ways to help myself. Soon after he was born, I was burned out and had to quit working at the other two locations. In the intervening years since I graduated from SCNM, I have built my practice and now have two sons, ages five and seven. My methods have not only helped cure me, but many patients.

In the last ten years, I have created this protocol called *Seven Steps to Heal Your Thyroid* based on my personal struggle with this condition and that of my patients. After following this plan, I began feeling like myself again, but my hypothyroidism could have been treated sooner.

I would have had this problem since I was a teenager. I remember being the heavy one in school, even though I never ate as much as my friends did. I never knew when to expect my menstrual cycles since they were always irregular, and I could skip couple months between them sometimes. My hair was dry and brittle and would fall out easily. My symptoms kept getting worse as I grew up, but nobody would address this in India, and it goes undiagnosed in the United States as well. This has increased my passion for helping others heal their thyroid. Because of my unique condition, I understand the patients who have hypothyroidism and keep getting referrals from the people I have helped. It has become my mission to serve and help people feel like themselves again.

I know how people push themselves past their limit every day and just try to be normal people in society. How tired we can be, how much we struggle with losing weight, and the low feelings that are there each day. The depression. I have been there, but we don't have to feel this way. With the seven steps, I'm going to demonstrate how everyone can feel rejuvenated once more.

I have created these seven steps for everyone to feel like themselves again while increasing their energy, elevating their mood and optimizing their weight.

Life is simple. Life can be simple again.

STEP 1:

UNDERSTANDING YOUR THYROID

The thyroid gland might not be a part of the body people think of often. We know about the heart, lungs, and brain, but how much do we know about the thyroid, besides perhaps hearing it mentioned on our favorite medical show? Yet the thyroid plays a significant role in overall health, but thyroid problems often go undiagnosed.

This butterfly-shaped organ, located in the neck region by the larynx, or Adam's apple, produces the hormones that regulate the body's metabolism. It is considered the master gland for metabolism and its function affects every organ and cell in the body. Thus, when the thyroid is slow, everything is slow. One could have a slow heart rate causing low energy, slow GI function leading to constipation, and slow brain function leading to foggy thinking, unable to concentrate, and depression. The decrease in metabolism makes it difficult for one to lose weight or gain weight easily, even though they don't eat much. Thus, in order to increase energy, elevate the mood, and optimize weight, understanding how the thyroid gland works is essential.

The pituitary gland is the master gland of the body and is located below the hypothalamus in the brain. It sends a signal in the form of TSH (Thyroid Stimulating Hormone) to the thyroid gland to stimulate it to produce thyroid hormones. The thyroid gland responds to this signal by making T4 (Thyroxine) hormone. The body then converts this T4 to T3 (Triiodothyronine), which is considered the active thyroid hormone that the cells utilize, and in turn, produce energy (Bunevicius, et al., 1999).

To illustrate the function of the thyroid, I would like to welcome you to my office.

Let's compare the human body to the office in which I work. My office is comfortable and well taken care of, much like how the human body should function, cleanly and efficiently. After you walk through the doors, the Arizona sun shining behind you, you will meet the smiling secretaries, which in the case of your body, represent your thyroid. They help keep the clinic running, like how your thyroid keeps your body running well. The messages they handle are like the hormones Triiodothyronine (T3) and Thyroxine (T4). I would then be the pituitary gland, the master gland, as I instruct them about scheduling and more. Yet I must adhere to the rules of the clinic or hypothalamus.

If any part of this functioning system becomes unbalanced, like the messages I must send to the secretaries as they manage the front desk, patients' schedules would become a mess, appointments would be missed, and the clinic would slow down or go out of business. The functioning system would no longer work or simply slow down, the same way the thyroid can slow down.

THYROID DISORDERS

Hypothyroidism vs. Hyperthyroidism

In this book, I am mostly going to talk about hypothyroidism. One in every five women is diagnosed with this condition. One of the most common reasons for hypothyroidism is Hashimoto's Thyroiditis. While hypothyroidism is a condition in which your thyroid gland is under producing thyroid hormones, hyperthyroidism is a condition in which the thyroid gland is over producing the thyroid hormones. Even though thyroid cancer is rare, these days, we hear about it quite often. Have you wondered why? I am going to leave that topic to another specialist who focuses in oncology. My aim for this book is to educate about hypothyroidism, what is causing it to be so common and how we approach the treatment.

Imagine crawling into the doctor's office, the lights bright in your tired eyes. You would rather be at home, curled up in your cozy comforter. You haven't been sleeping well and just need a nap. But that's why you're there, sitting in the clean room trying to find out where your energy has gone, why you have such brittle hair, and why your mind has been in such a fog. You wrap up in your sweater and wait for the doctor, wondering when you will feel normal again.

Your doctor seems to understand and runs lab tests to find out what is the cause of you feeling this way. He wants to test all your hormone levels and see if they are unbalanced or are too low. Hypothyroidism, he tells you, is a condition where there are low levels of thyroid hormone in the body. The symptoms can range from fatigue, weight gain, dry skin and hair, constipation, depression, brain fogginess or difficulty concentrating, sleep problems, hair loss, feeling cold easily or cold intolerance, and menstrual irregularities.

You wait for the results, and they come back with a positive diagnosis of hypothyroidism. Shocked, you wonder how this happened. You learn the leading cause of hypothyroidism is Hashimoto's Thyroiditis. Though you were tested before, your hormone levels were always within "normal" range.

And then you find out that you could have been tested for Hashimoto's Thyroiditis earlier, and you may have struggled with the signs and symptoms of hypothyroidism for decades. It went undiagnosed because doctors don't usually test for the thyroid antibodies, though they can easily be checked via bloodwork when ordering the other thyroid tests. Many doctors treat the thyroid according to the TSH levels only, which can be wide-ranging. You were finally diagnosed purely based on numbers. Yet, I look to treat the person rather than the just the lab work.

I went through a similar situation where I could have been diagnosed earlier in life for my own thyroid condition. In my teens, it was very difficult for me to lose weight. My friends didn't have a problem with it, but I always struggled, even though I ate much less compared to them and I would still gain weight. My hair would be thin and be falling out, and my menstrual cycles were always irregular or even missing for two months in a row. All of this showed I had an underlying thyroid condition that was always there. It was never picked up or noticed by my family or doctors. I realized this only much later in life after all of these problems went away upon correcting my thyroid function. This happens to so many women, and one way to prevent this is to know more about the thyroid and Hashimoto's Thyroiditis.

The words hypothyroidism and hyperthyroidism are very similar, one small change from the "o" to "er" makes a big difference. Hypothyroidism is under-production of thyroid hormones while hyperthyroidism is over production; it produces too much of the thyroid hormones. A simple way to think of this is like a hyper child. You have "hyper" thyroid rather than a sleepy one.

Symptoms of hyperthyroidism include increased heart rate, heart palpitations (when the heart feels like it skips a beat), anxiety, jitteriness, and loss of weight. Everything becomes fast rather than slow. It is really quite the opposite of hypothyroidism, where the body and function slow down, and you gain weight.

Hashimoto's Thyroiditis

In the last ten years of my clinical practice, I have seen a steady rise in the diagnosis of hypothyroidism. Hashimoto's Thyroiditis is a common cause of hypothyroidism. I would like to explain how this happens.

Hashimoto's is an auto immune condition in which the body forms antibodies that attack its own thyroid gland and suppress its activity. These antibodies cause inflammation on the thyroid gland. If it goes untreated, this inflammation will destroy the gland eventually, making it impossible for your thyroid to produce the hormones you need and will ultimately cause hypothyroidism.

Hashimoto's is a complicated condition with many layers that need to be unraveled. While conventional medicine looks at each body system as a separate category and is only concerned with the thyroid's ability to produce thyroid hormones,

Hashimoto's is more than just hypothyroidism and should be looked at and treated separately.

When someone is diagnosed with Hashimoto's and the antibodies are fluctuating, one can experience alternating symptoms, from hyperthyroidism to hypothyroidism. It's a roller coaster of symptoms and hormone levels. It can make it very difficult to control the thyroid treatment when the patient goes between hypothyroidism and hyperthyroidism. Because of this fluctuation, I tell my patients to inform me if they start noticing heart palpitations, jitteriness, anxiety, and difficulty sleeping. These symptoms would indicate that they are getting too much of the thyroid medicine and their dose will have to be adjusted.

From what I've seen, in the case of Hashimoto's, these fluctuations will eventually stop and become just hypothyroidism. It's only in the initial stages of Hashimoto's that the hormones can fluctuate this way. However, there are still separate instances when a person can have just hyperthyroidism as well. Our bodies keep a fine balance, a sort of dance between the body parts, with the thyroid being the choreographer.

Hypothyroidism, Hashimoto's Thyroiditis and sometimes Hyperthyroidism are the thyroid problems I encounter and treat daily.

I would like to discuss two of these now. First is when a patient is making enough T4 hormone, but the body is unable to convert it to its active form, T3. A few influences preventing this crucial conversion are being advanced in age, overeating goitrogen (kale, cauliflower, brussel sprouts), your stress, taking certain medications, chemotherapy or radiation exposure, toxin exposure, extreme exercise, inflammation, low iron, and low testosterone. Once the problem is diagnosed, it can be treated appropriately. Second is molecular mimicry, which I will discuss next.

MOLECULAR MIMICRY

What happens in molecular mimicry is that we have these protein sequences and antigens. The antibodies bind to the specific protein sequences of antigens. While gluten, casein, and your tissues may all be different, they share some of the same protein sequences. A cross-reaction occurs when your immune system cannot distinguish between these molecules. Gluten (wheat, barley, rye, oats, related species, and hybrids and products of these) and casein, the main protein found in milk, may be different, but they share the same sequences. They "mimic" each other. There is a cross-reaction since the immune system may not be able to distinguish between the antibodies and they attack the thyroid gland. This is how molecular mimicry causes Hashimoto's Thyroiditis.

Molecular mimicry also happens with halogens (chlorine, bromine, iodine, and fluorine). The body is exposed to these from different sources, and some of those are toxic. Out of all 4 of them, Iodine is an essential mineral for the formation of the thyroid hormone while the others are not. But due to their similar structure, the body confuses other halogens with iodine and causes a cross-reaction on the thyroid gland.

MOLECULAR MIMICRY

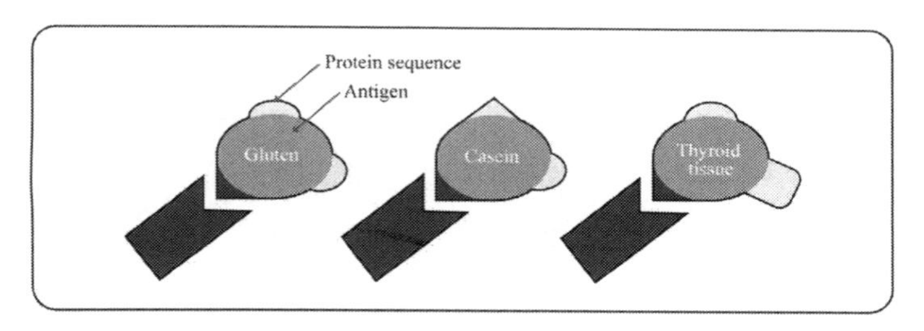

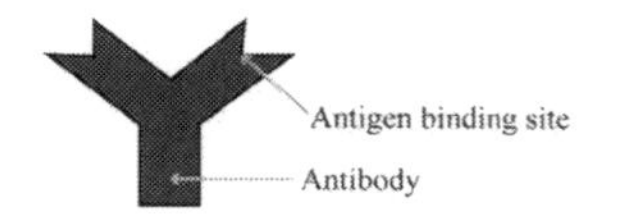

Antibodies bind to the specific protein sequences of antigens. While gluten, casein, and your own tissues may all be different, they share some of the same protein sequences. A cross reaction occurs when your immune system cannot distinguish between these molecules.

Offending Agents to the Thyroid

It is good to know the offending agents, or things that cause harm to your thyroid, so you can avoid them and possibly prevent a problem in the future. A few are gluten, heavy metals, and HPA-Axis insufficiency, which has to do with adrenal imbalances. Certain medications can also affect the thyroid such as Amiodarone, beta blockers, Dilantin, Prednisone, synthetic progesterones, and Lithium, especially if taken with a thyroid medication..

APPROPRIATE THYROID TESTING

The first step to a healthy thyroid is finding a correct diagnosis, and the earlier we find the problem, the better we can treat it. There are some important tests that doctors can ask for to check thyroid function. Blood tests, as well as thyroid ultrasounds, are used to diagnose thyroid disorders.

TSH (Thyroid Stimulating Hormone) Test

What is TSH again?

TSH, or thyroid-stimulating hormone, is produced by the pituitary gland. TSH is what tells the thyroid to produce the T4 hormone. T4 then needs to be converted to T3, which is the active thyroid hormone that makes body systems work optimally, to not be slow as I mentioned earlier. The cells utilize the T3 and produce energy. The signal from TSH to the thyroid gland works on a negative feedback loop, meaning if thyroid hormone production is low, the TSH is stimulated to work harder and therefore tests higher than normal. On the other hand, if the TSH tests lower than normal, it means that the thyroid gland is over-producing the thyroid hormones. Therefore, high TSH means hypothyroidism and low TSH means hyperthyroidism.

TSH is generally considered the standard test for thyroid. However, I have found it to be an unreliable test and consider it more of a screening test because numerous times when I have tested TSH on my patients, it comes back fine when they are complaining of hypothyroid symptoms. They have seen a number of doctors prior to me, who have sent them away saying that everything is fine and they don't need any treatment. I have listened to these patients and ordered a complete thyroid panel, which has given me a clear picture of their thyroid function. My complete thyroid panel includes TSH, T3, FT3, T4, FT4, Anti-thyroglobulin and Thyroid Peroxidase Antibodies.

Lab ranges of TSH are from 0.4 to 4.5. This is a very wide range. Ideal TSH levels should be close or less than one.

Free T3 and Free T4 Tests

The Free T3 and Free T4 tests measure the T3 and T4 that are freely available in the blood and unattached to proteins. Since certain conditions such as pregnancy and liver disease can increase carrier protein concentrations, doctors will have a more precise reading by assessing the levels of free T3 and T4.

- Free Thyroxine FT4 tests measure the levels of thyroxine in the blood, since a low level could indicate hypothyroidism.

- Free Iodothyronine FT3 tests measure the levels of triiodothyronine in the blood, since a low level could also mean hypothyroidism.

Let me explain the reason behind ordering all these tests. The T3 hormone is bound to a protein while FT3 is freely circulating in the blood, similarly for the T4 and FT4. Sometimes the T4 levels test out fine, but T3 levels are low. One probable reason could be that the body is not able to make the conversion from T4 to T3.

Maybe there are not enough nutrients that help this conversion. Perhaps it's the molecular mimicry that is causing Hashimoto's, or a sensitivity to gluten. Environment could be a factor as well, combined with toxin exposure.

From a thyroid treatment standpoint, this helps, because if a patient is treated with Synthroid or Levothyroxine, which is the usual standard of care, it provides them the synthetically prepared T4 hormone alone. If the person is unable to convert this over to T3, which is the biologically active hormone, then their physician would know based on the levels of T3 tested that they may need to adjust their treatment and probably add a medication that provides the T3 hormone also. I will address the choice of medications in the following chapter.

Thyroid Antibody Tests

(Thyroid peroxidase and Antithyroglobulin Antibodies)

The immune system produces antibodies to protect us from foreign invaders.

Antibodies are produced by white blood cells (lymphocytes) to destroy harmful attackers such as bacteria or viruses. People who have Hashimoto's Thyroiditis produce either one or both of these antibodies that attack the thyroid gland. It could be due to molecular mimicry that was explained above. One of the reasons for developing Hashimoto's is "leaky gut." There is a chapter dedicated to your gut health in this book.

In most cases of Hashimoto's Thyroiditis, blood tests will reveal one or two types of anti-thyroid antibodies. TPO is the most common antibody present (in up to 95% of those with Hashimoto's), and often antibodies against Thyroglobulin (TG) are found as well (around 80%).

These antibodies may appear decades before a change in TSH is detected, thus allowing people to make an intervention before the thyroid gland gets damaged to a point where it will no longer be able to make enough thyroid hormone. In this book, you will learn about the different causes that lead to this condition and how we can prevent it by using appropriate natural treatments. An ounce of prevention is worth a pound of a cure.

This is why it is so important to check for Hashimoto's. By applying correct testing methods, we can properly treat and possibly prevent hypothyroidism. It is my mission to treat the person rather than treat the lab values. Understanding the tests and lab values will help me to treat the whole person.

Thyroid Ultrasounds

An order is given to do a Thyroid ultrasound and is performed at an imaging center. Ultrasound imaging involves the use of a small transducer (probe) and ultrasound gel placed directly on the skin over the thyroid gland. High-frequency sound waves are transmitted from the probe through the gel into the body. It is used to capture the size, structure, and any pathological lesion. When the thyroid gland is enlarged, it is referred to as a goiter and suggests hypothyroidism. When a person has Hashimoto's Thyroiditis, more blood flow is seen over the thyroid gland, suggesting inflammation.

I had a patient whose thyroid gland was 90% destroyed. She had Hashimoto's undiagnosed for so many decades that her thyroid gland was damaged and was evident on the thyroid ultrasound. The ultrasound is what finally determined the need for a high dose of thyroid medication for her. Even though her thyroid gland was not surgically removed, which would naturally indicate a need for a high dose of the medication, it was as good as not being there since it was destroyed by her chronic Hashimoto's. While I don't order thyroid ultrasounds for every person, they can be beneficial, depending on the person's individual need.

Another thing doctors look for is thyroid nodules. These nodules are hard to feel by external palpation, but the thyroid ultrasound can pick them up if they are there. If the nodule is big, they will typically have to be biopsied to check to see if it is cancerous. It is a scary thought; however, you can feel a little calmer knowing that 95 percent of the time, they are benign, meaning non-cancerous.

The rest of the tests that I would like to mention here are blood tests, which I do order for all my patients. The patient is given a lab slip to take to a lab for a blood draw.

Optimal vs. Normal Thyroid Levels

After the blood is drawn, the results would then come back to me. There is a wide range of results for the thyroid hormones. A patient can be a point away from not being within the optimal ranges, which is vast, and be told they are fine, even though they have all these symptoms that go with a thyroid problem. So, if you fall within the lab results' "normal" or healthy ranges, this does not mean that you have optimal thyroid levels. There is a huge difference between normal and optimal ranges.

These are the levels I personally look for when reading a lab result.

- TSH: 1 or less
- T3: 130+
- T4: 8 +
- FT3: 3.5 +
- FT4: 1-1.5

Thyroid Antibodies - should not be elevated.

Be aware when looking at results that lab ranges will vary from country to country or from lab to lab. Make sure you are closer to mid to higher range. If you are closer to the lower end, you may have subclinical hypothyroidism.

WHERE TO START?

It can all be a little much to start with and can feel overwhelming, but this is why I want to give you a few ways you can begin to heal your thyroid right away, and thus increase your energy, elevate your mood, and optimize your weight.

For this first chapter, though we've discussed a lot, the answer is a bit simple. This chapter was all about understanding the role of the thyroid gland, and if you have symptoms, understanding which tests are needed to get a correct diagnosis. If you feel you may have a thyroid condition, check with your doctor. Or, if your thyroid levels have come back normal, but you still have symptoms, find a Naturopathic Doctor like me so that I can run comprehensive lab tests on you and help find the underlying problem. You don't need to struggle every day. A correct diagnosis is the first step towards optimal thyroid health.

STEP 2:

NATUROPATHIC TREATMENTS

I am a Naturopathic Doctor, so the six Naturopathic Principles have a close meaning to my heart. I always keep these in mind when I see a patient.

1. The Healing Power of Nature

Trust in the body's inherent wisdom to heal itself.

2. Identify and Treat the Causes

Look beyond the symptoms to the underlying cause.

3. First Do No Harm

Utilize the most natural, least invasive and least toxic therapies.

4. Doctor as Teacher

Educate patients on the steps to achieving and maintaining health.

5. Treat the Whole Person

View the body as an integrated whole in all its physical and spiritual dimensions.

6. Prevention

Focus on overall health, wellness and disease prevention.

The human body has an innate ability to heal itself. The healing comes from within. If you get a minor cut on your finger or arm, you don't run off to the hospital. The body will trigger its own healing process, and without you doing anything at all, it will heal itself.

At times, when the body is unable to complete the process of healing, Naturopathic Doctors can provide some supportive treatments. If you rub some Arnica gel or Homeopathic Calendula ointment on that minor cut, it will enhance the healing. Similarly, when the thyroid slows down or speeds up, by providing some natural treatments, it can correct itself. This small example shows how a Naturopathic Doctor treats their patients. As a whole.

One of the six fundamental principles of Naturopathic Medicine states how we must identify and treat the root cause, not just the symptoms. If a patient has chronic headaches, I wouldn't want to simply give them a pain reliever and send them home, but instead look at their emotional health, diet, and other areas to find the source of their pain. For me, the problem was Hashimoto's. Yet there was a point when I tried to follow principle number one and let my body heal itself, but eventually, it needed treatment.

After I gave birth to my first child, we had a wonderful vacation in Hawaii, a dream. I don't know if it was the relaxing sun or the sand on my feet that caused my good mood and created thoughts that I didn't need any more support for my thyroid. I stopped taking my medication. After we came back from the trip, I immediately saw a change. I became exhausted once again and started having to push myself every day to complete simple tasks. I was producing less breast milk for my eight-month-old. No matter what I tried with my diet and pumping, I couldn't produce more milk for my son, which is another indication of hypothyroidism. I was driving back from work one day and started to fall asleep at the wheel.

This was dangerous.

I knew I had to accept that something had been helping my body and that I had to correct this deficiency again. In my case, my body couldn't heal itself; thus, I had to work on the Naturopathic

Principle number two and treat my condition. I needed to go back on my medication, and once I did, it was a night and day difference. I had my energy back,my pregnancy weight began to melt away, and I didn't have to struggle to wake up in the morning. This was because I decided to listen to my body and get the treatment needed.

Principle number four, Docere, or Doctor as Teacher, has a lot of meaning for me daily. I want to ensure my patients have a proper understanding of what their bodies are going through and what they can do to help themselves. You may hear someone talk about how knowledgeable their doctor is and, while this is an excellent recommendation to have, I want my patients to feel that they have become knowledgeable as well.

Through my own struggles with Hashimoto's, I had terrific mentors that helped me in my journey, like Dr. Tutera, whom I have previously mentioned. Dr. Thomas Kruzel is another mentor of mine who has had a major impact on my life and career. He is the owner of Rockwood Natural Medicine, where I worked from 2009-2018. When I first discovered I had a thyroid problem, I had elevated antibodies and all these symptoms of hypothyroidism, but my thyroid test results were "within normal ranges." He was the one who suggested Thytrophin PMG to help lower my thyroid antibodies and support my thyroid gland to function better. This has remained my very favorite thyroid supplement.

CHOICE OF PRESCRIPTION MEDICATIONS

The third Naturopathic Principle listed is to "do no harm." Therefore, once it is time to use a prescription medication for thyroid treatment, I want to make sure it is from the best natural sources and the safest for my patients.

Because of this, my first choice is Nature-Throid to correct hypothyroidism, which is the purest form of natural thyroid. It comes from the gland of the animal, so it's a natural source. The unique part about it is that it is a combination of the T4 and T3 hormones, unlike the plain T4 that comes in a synthetic version. It is very reasonably priced compared to other brands of thyroid medications. I see much better symptom improvement in my patients when I use Nature-Throid compared to synthetic thyroid medications. Some studies show there is improved cognitive performance, lowering of blood pressure, more energy, and improved lipid levels when using desiccated thyroid medications. Naturethroid and Armour Thyroid are both considered desiccated thyroid medications.

Armour Thyroid is another choice I use. It's made by a different company than Nature-Throid and has been around a long time, but it may have certain binders that Nature-Throid may not.

Levothyroxine is the most commonly prescribed thyroid medication. It is synthetic T4. Sometimes when patients with Hashimoto's start just on T4, they don't have much relief from their symptoms. Their dose gets increased repeatedly, but the problem is that their body is not converting the T4 they are receiving through the medication into the active hormone T3. Therefore, the addition of T3 really helps. Liothyronine is the synthetic T3 medication. With this combination of T4 +T3, the synthetic version works, and the patient's symptoms improve.

You may have heard rumors regarding thyroid medications and complications such as the two listed below, but these are myths.

Myth #1:
T3 is dangerous for your heart

Optimizing your thyroid improves cholesterol levels, decreases risk of congestive heart failure, and relaxes the blood vessels.. In fact, most patients with Advanced Congestive Heart Failure have altered Thyroid Metabolism.

- Subclinical hypothyroidism is linked with two times the risk of heart attack in women who are more than 55 years old.

Mild thyroid disease is a deep-rooted cardiac risk factor, like high cholesterol and smoking.

Myth #2:
Thyroid replacement causes osteoporosis

There is no decrease in BMD (Bone Mineral Density) in pre or post menopausal women receiving thyroid treatment. Also, high-dose thyroid does not appear to be a significant risk factor for osteoporosis.

Do not let rumors affect your decision. Optimal functioning of your thyroid is an essential aspect of staying healthy. If you have any concerns regarding myths or rumors, you should always discuss them with your doctor.

BOTANICAL MEDICINE

Herbs for Hypothyroidism

Another way to heal your thyroid is by using botanical medicine.

Ashwagandha

Ashwagandha is known as an adaptogenic herb. Adaptogenic herbs help patients adapt and deal with stress. They adapt to the need. Thus, it would help in both hypothyroid and hyperthyroid conditions by optimizing the thyroid hormone production. In Ayurvedic medicine, the literal Indian meaning of its name is "smell of the horse." I think about it like this: when you take this herb, you will feel the horsepower!

Kelp

Kelp is one food that is rich in iodine. Iodine is one of the minerals required for the formation of the thyroid hormone. It is a brown type of seaweed which people have used when traditional medications have not worked in fighting thyroid issues. Kelp can either be eaten raw or it can be consumed in the form of teas and supplements.

Fucus

Fucus vesiculosus, also known as bladder wrack, is primarily used to enhance thyroid function in cases of goiter and as an aid in weight loss for obesity. It is a good source of iodine.

Siberian Ginseng

This herb works well for those who have an underactive thyroid. It helps to give the body energy, which makes it perfect for addressing the fatigue that often accompanies low thyroid function. Siberian ginseng is a gentle stimulant that will give you that boost of energy you want.

Nettle

It is often referred to as stinging nettle and is a perfect thyroid tonic, as it offers a balance between those suffering from an underactive thyroid or an overactive thyroid.

Herbs for Hyperthyroidism

When someone with hyperthyroidism or Graves' Disease follows a natural treatment protocol, the obvious goal is to restore their health back to normal. However, initially, it is essential for the person to manage their hyperthyroid symptoms.

Bugleweed

Bugleweed acts like a natural antithyroid herb. Clinical studies have shown that it inhibits T4 output. Pharmacological studies show that in addition to decreasing T4 levels, people that take bugleweed have decreased T3 levels, most likely due to it inhibiting the conversion of T4 to T3.

Motherwort

Motherwort has numerous functions, one of which is that it works as a natural beta blocker, meaning it helps to lower the fast-ended heart rate. People with hyperthyroidism have an increased heart rate (tachycardia) and heart palpitations due to increase in production of the thyroid hormones. This herb has antithyroid activity.

Lemon Balm

Similar to motherwort, lemon balm has numerous functions. With regard to hyperthyroidism and Graves' Disease, it inhibits TSH, which in turn can help to reduce the excessive secretion of thyroid hormone.

HOMEOPATHIC MEDICINES

Homeopathy is an art and science. It is a medicine that is based on the philosophy that like cures like. Thus, to find the best medicine for a person, a Naturopathic Physician must match the symptoms of the person to the medication that has been proved prior with similar symptoms. The following is a list of medicines that have been most helpful in patients with thyroid disorders.

Iodum

This medicine will help patients with a hard goiter who have a sensation of constriction. They may have swelling and induration of the cervical glands. It works in people with dark hair and eyes who are emaciated, and those who sweat easily.

Calcarea Carb

This works for people with painless enlargement of glands and who are prone to glandular enlargements in general, beyond the thyroid gland. It works in people who are fair, overweight, and flabby, who get easily tired with much sweating, cold extremities, and sour smell of the body. They also tend towards obesity.

Phytolacca

This helps people with a nodulated goiter. Glands of the right side of the neck are swollen. The patient experiences shooting pains that are worse in the damp weather and at night. It works for people who are emaciated, with a pale and sunken face. They are usually exhausted and are prone to rheumatism.

Spongia

A candidate for this medicine is prone to goiter, thyroid glands swollen with suffocative paroxysms, or spasms, at night. They get cold easily and may feel as if they're breathing through a sponge. It works mostly for women and children having light hair and fair complexion.

Thyroidinum

This is made from a dried gland of sheep or calf. A state of puffiness and obesity may be regarded as a keynote indication for this medicine. These people crave sweets and have a thirst for cold water. They are also sensitive to cold.

NUTRITION AT THE CORE OF PERSONALIZED WELLNESS

Yet, before we even treat the patient with prescriptions, botanical medicines, herbs, and homeopathic medicines, we must look at their nutrition. If possible, prevention is essential. One possible way to prevent a thyroid problem, or at least keep it at bay for a while, is through adequate nutrition, which can be checked through a micronutrient test.

Micronutrient Testing

One of the tools that helps me find out what your thyroid gland may need to heal is the micronutrient test.

Wouldn't it be nice if you could just know which supplement your body needs so you don't have to take so many? With micronutrient testing, this is possible.

Micronutrients are vitamins and minerals required in small quantities that are essential to your health. In fact, your internal body works on a complex maze of biochemical pathways. These biochemical reactions take place inside your cells and are responsible for all the bodily functions to happen optimally. Micronutrients are required in various stages of these biochemical reactions.

"Overwhelming evidence suggests that a lack of these vital nutrients has a profound impact on the body's immune system. Thus, adequate intake of these vitamins and minerals could mean the difference between a healthy life and a life fraught with disease" (Barman, 2014-2016, para. 2). In order for your thyroid gland to produce adequate hormones, certain nutrients are essential. Please refer to the picture provided by SpectraCell Laboratories that explains this.

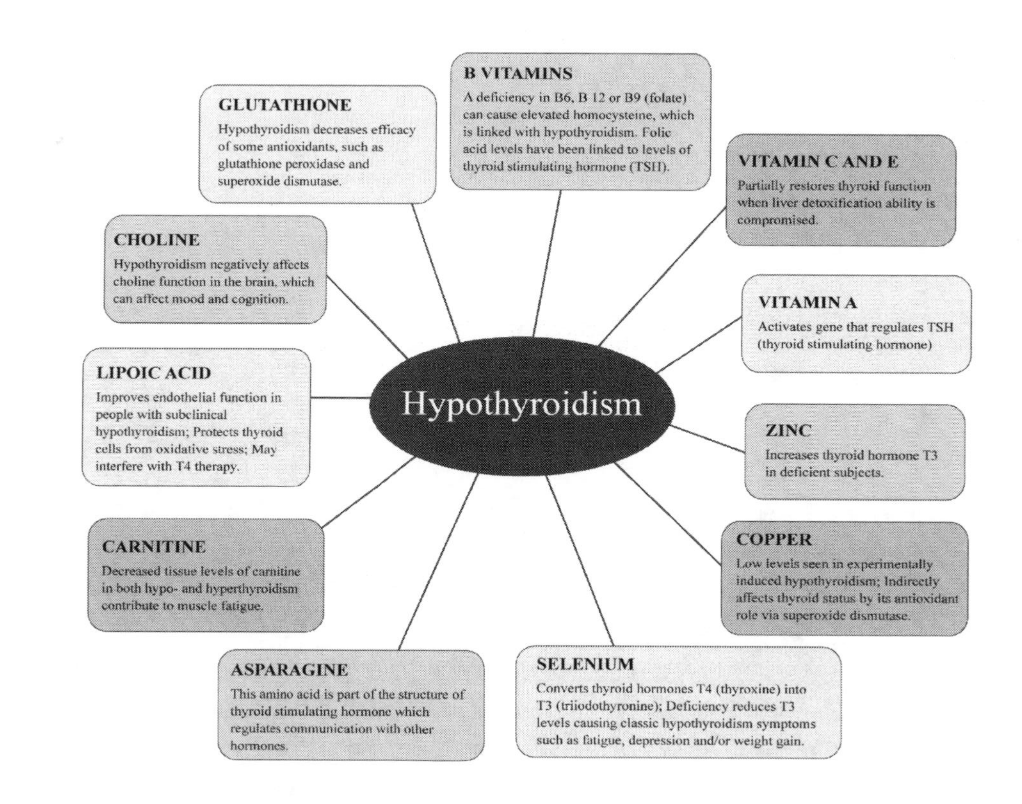
Hypothyroidism
GLUTATHIONE
Hypothyroidism decreases efficacy of some antioxidants, such as glutathione peroxidase and superoxide dismutase.
B VITAMINS
A deficiency in B6, B 12 or B9 (folate) can cause elevated homocysteine, which is linked with hypothyroidism. Folic acid levels have been linked to levels of thyroid stimulating hormone (TSH).
VITAMIN C AND E
Partially restores thyroid function when liver detoxification ability is compromised.
CHOLINE
Hypothyroidism negatively affects choline function in the brain, which can affect mood and cognition.
VITAMIN A
Activates gene that regulates TSH (thyroid stimulating hormone)
LIPOIC ACID
Improves endothelial function in people with subclinical hypothyroidism; Protects thyroid cells from oxidative stress; May interfere with T4 therapy.
ZINC
Increases thyroid hormone T3 in deficient subjects.
CARNITINE
Decreased tissue levels of carnitine in both hypo- and hyperthyroidism contribute to muscle fatigue.
COPPER
Low levels seen in experimentally induced hypothyroidism; Indirectly affects thyroid status by its antioxidant role via superoxide dismutase.
ASPARAGINE
This amino acid is part of the structure of thyroid stimulating hormone which regulates communication with other hormones.
SELENIUM
Converts thyroid hormones T4 (thyroxine) into T3 (triiodothyronine); Deficiency reduces T3 levels causing classic hypothyroidism symptoms such as fatigue, depression and/or weight gain.

SpectraCell's exclusive Micronutrient Test is a comprehensive nutritional analysis of the body's intracellular function. It measures 35 selected vitamins, minerals, antioxidants, and other essential micronutrients within the white blood cells. This analysis can reveal a person's functional nutritional status over a much longer period of time than conventional static serum testing.

In order to accomplish this, blood is drawn and sent to the lab, where they grow the white blood cells for three weeks. It's an intracellular look at these white blood cells, upon which the report of the micronutrient status is regenerated. They provide a nice report, both graphically and numerically, which is easy for the patient to understand. The report not only shows what the patient may be deficient in and by how much, but also provides a repletion protocol plus how to correct this deficiency with food choices. I show a sample report to my patients so they can understand what to expect from doing this test.

For example, a sample report will show that a patient requires oleic acid, glutathione, and vitamin E, and even how much of each nutrient is necessary so then they may take them through a supplement. Dietary sources of these nutrients are also mentioned. Thus, the person can make food choices that are rich in these nutrients. Based on the result of the micronutrient test, I can correct nutrient deficiencies in my patients and personalize their treatments.

I had a micronutrient test performed during the initial stages of my thyroid problem and found out I had three deficiencies. I started supplementing those and felt much better. It gave me some justification and a feeling that it was possible to correct this problem. In some patients, I have seen life-changing results by simply correcting their nutrient deficiencies.

I had one patient in her teens who did not want to do anything except sleep, since she felt exhausted and had joint pains. Based on her micronutrient test results, we were able to correct her nutrient status. She was then able to get up and do things. Her mom personally came to thank me since she saw her daughter jump, move, and excited about life after more than five years.

So now let's talk about the nutrients that are essential for proper thyroid functioning. You saw from the picture by SpectraCell that many nutrients play a role in appropriate thyroid functioning, and the best way to find out what your cells need is via a micronutrient test. Yet I have five supplements that I commonly suggest to my patients with hypothyroidism and Hashimoto's Thyroiditis.

Thytrophin PMG

Prevention of disease is important and is one of the six fundamental principles. If a patient is in the early diagnosis of hypothyroidism or showing positive thyroid antibodies, and the thyroid tests are within normal ranges, but the patient is presenting with symptoms of hypothyroidism, I would start them on Thytrophin PMG. Thytrophin PMG is a whole food-based supplement made by Standard Process, which is an almost 100-year-old supplement company. It uses DNA and RNA extracted from the gland of the animal. What it does is it helps to lower the thyroid antibodies. It's a useful supplement that I used when I was diagnosed with Hashimoto's. Thytrophin PMG helps during molecular mimicry because it will attach to the antibodies and reduce the numbers. The starting dose is usually two tablets per day with food.

Selenium

Selenium is required for the conversion of the T4 to the T3. If you remember, T3 is the active thyroid hormone that the cells utilize to produce energy. Sometimes we will run the thyroid panel and the T4 seems fine, but the T3 is low. Deficiency of selenium causes classic hypothyroid symptoms such as fatigue, depression, and weight gain. The best dietary source of selenium is Brazil nuts. Eat a handful of these as a snack every day. Otherwise, it can be taken in a supplement form called Selenomethionine in doses about 200 micrograms per day. Vitamin E, 400 IUs, if taken with selenium, helps to facilitate its absorption.

B Vitamins

A deficiency in B6, B12, or B9 (folate) can cause elevated homocysteine, which is linked to hypothyroidism. Elevated homocysteine levels can cause increased inflammation, irritation of the blood vessels, heart disease, neurological problems, and other symptoms. B vitamins play a vital role in different biochemical pathways of the body and are essential for numerous bodily functions, including the thyroid. I recommend the use of an active B complex to be taken daily with food.

Glutathione

Hypothyroidism decreases the efficacy of some antioxidants, such as glutathione peroxidase and superoxide dismutase. Antioxidants are needed to kill the free radicals that are generated due to oxidative stress. Therefore, it is essential to have good levels of this "master antioxidant."

Glutathione is found in every cell of the body and plays an essential roles in protein synthesis, synthesis and repair of DNA, enzyme function, transport, and cell maturation. Optimal levels of glutathione have been associated with physical and mental health. The highest concentration of glutathione is found in the liver, where it offers antioxidant support, protects tissue and maintains detoxification. Liposomal Glutathione or Nrf2 are supplements that I recommend to increase glutathione levels. Glutathione is also available in

IV injectable and transdermal forms.

Iron

Adequate levels of iron are important for thyroid function. Many women that come to see me test deficient for iron and this does affect their thyroid hormone production. Serum Ferritin is an accurate way to check for iron levels. It is a simple blood test done by a regular lab.

Most of the iron supplements that are available in the market cause constipation. I would choose a form of iron that is easily absorbed and is non-constipating. I recommend Ferrasorb, which is a complete blood-building formula with folate B12 and iron supplement. It provides the active forms of vitamin B12 (adenosylcobalamin and methylcobalamin) and folate (folinic acid and 5MTHF) and includes well-absorbed non-constipating iron picolinate. If you prefer a liquid form, try Floradix, which is a plant-based iron that also works well.

Sometimes the food we eat doesn't have all the nutrients that we need; therefore, supplements are helpful to give us those nutrients. Many times, patients who have Hashimoto's don't require medication to start with, but they may benefit from using a thyroid supplement to help the thyroid gland to work better. These supplements, with help from your doctor, may help treat underlying causes of thyroid problems and help you feel like yourself again.

The delivery of the nutrients can be oral or via a nutrient IV. While both ways of administering these supplements are effective, the nutrient IV has some advantages over the pill or oral method. The nutrient IV is great because it can be customized for each patient based on their micronutrient test results. The nutrients are administered directly into the bloodstream, and this way, the patient can tolerate much higher doses of the beneficial nutrients without adverse effects.

For example, if beyond five grams of Vitamin C is taken orally, it can cause loose stools and diarrhea, but through an IV, 25 grams can be given safely without any problems. The IV also has the advantage of the nutrients being able to reach the cells and nourish them. But when supplements are taken in a pill form, a lot of it is flushed out in the urine.

Dr. Isabella Wentz, popularly known as the Thyroid Pharmacist, has been doing some excellent work in spreading awareness and educating people about Hashimoto's Thyroiditis.

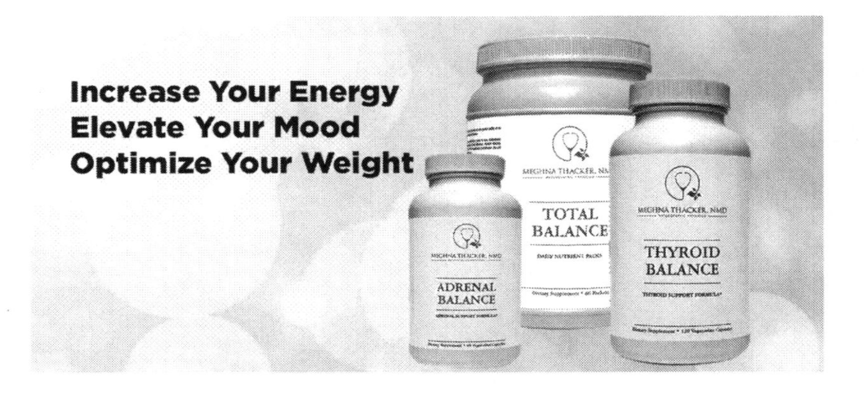

I am very excited to Introduce You to 3 of my Formulas that will support your Thyroid, Adrenal & Over-all Health.

All Dr. Meghna Thacker, PLLC Formulas Meet or Exceed cGMP Quality Standards and are available to purchase through my website, www.meghnathacker.com

Thyroid Balance

Clinical Applications

- Supports Healthy Thyroid Function*
- Supports the Body's Conversion of T4 to the More Active Hormone T3*

Thyroid Balance features targeted nutrients and herbs that support healthy thyroid hormone biosynthesis. This combination may facilitate the expression of thyroid hormone genes. The addition of ashwagandha and guggul extract may aid in the conversion of thyroxine to triiodothyronine (T4 to T3) and may assist in maintaining healthy blood lipid levels already within the normal range.*

Adrenal Balance

Clinical Applications

- Promotes Energy Production and Stamina*
- Supports the Body's Adaptogenic Response*
- Supports the Body's Response to Stress*
- Promotes Adrenal Physiological Functions*

Adrenal Balance features a comprehensive blend of nutrients and botanical extracts targeted to supporting the body's adaptogenic response to promote optimal energy production, stamina, and the management of everyday stressors. Adrenal glandular tissue, sourced from Argentinian bovine to safeguard purity, rounds out the ingredient profile.*

Total Balance

Clinical Applications

- Provide Foundation Micronutrition for a Variety of Protocols*
- Support Improved Dietary Nutrient Intake*
- Provide Antioxidant Support*

Total Balance is a convenient way to get daily comprehensive nutritional support. Each daily dose packet contains several different supplements that provide Albion® chelated minerals; activated B vitamins, including 5-MTHF as Quatrefolic® and methylcobalamin as MecobalActiveTM; botanicals for antioxidant protection; and fresh, pure, third-party assayed fish oils.

*These statements have not been evaluated by the Food and Drug Administration. This product is not intended to diagnose, treat, cure, or prevent any disease.

Thyroid Healing Foods

On my Facebook Page, Dr. Meghna Thacker, you can keep an eye out for Foods that Heal your Thyroid Recipes. There, you will find even more useful tips. I also recommend the book Thyroid Healing by Anthony Williams. In it, he mentions Thyroid Grab & Go Combos, ex: cauliflower florets + apple slices together bring down inflammation on your thyroid. Another one is kale + mango; this combination of alkaloids & carotenes allows them to easily enter the thyroid and stop the growth of nodules and cysts there.

Here is a list of foods for you to incorporate into your diet. You can write them on a paper and stick it on your fridge. It will remind you to use them when you are preparing your meals.

List of Thyroid Healing Foods	
Artichokes	Aloe Vera
Apples	Arugula
Asparagus	Avocados
Bananas	Basil
Berries	Cauliflower
Celery	Cilantro
Coconut Oil	Cucumbers
Dates	Fennel
Figs	Garlic
Ginger	Hemp Seeds
Kale	Lemons & Limes
Lettuce	Mangoes
Maple Syrup	Nuts (walnuts, brazil nuts, almonds, and cashews)
Onions	Oranges & Tangerines
Papayas	Parsley
Pears	Pomegranates
Potatoes	Radishes
Raw Honey	Sesame Seeds
Spinach	Sprouts & Microgreens
Squash	Sweet Potatoes
Thyme	Tomatoes
Turmeric	

WHERE TO START?

Once you have been diagnosed with a thyroid problem, you must begin by doing a micronutrient test to help you discover what nutrients your cells need to function optimally. I have seen cases where merely treating the deficiency with nutrients, orally or through an IV, has changed a patient's life.

The next step is to talk to your doctor about your treatment and medication options. Discuss botanical and homeopathic medicine choices. Consider Nature-Throid or a desiccated thyroid as a choice of medication, if needed.

And yet, sometimes patients may not even need to start with a prescription. If you're still in the early stages of Hashimoto's or hypothyroidism, you may want to use my favorite supplement, Thytrophin PMG, just like I did.

STEP 3: HEAL YOUR GUT

What did you eat today?

In Naturopathic Medicine, we believe that disease originates in the gut (gastro-intestinal tract). Why do we believe this? Your gut is the seat to 80 % of your body's immunity. Since Hashimoto's is an autoimmune disorder, the health of your gut is vital. Many chronic diseases happen because of dysfunction of our immune system, ranging from rheumatoid arthritis to cancer. Thus, it makes sense when people say that the gut is the origin of most diseases.

But first, we must understand how each person is unique, not only with personalities but also unique from their genetic make-up. What makes us unique is our bio-individuality. Let me explain. What we eat is important, but what our gut can absorb and digest is what really matters. It all depends on your unique Gut Microbiome. Even if we all eat the same thing, I may react to a food differently than you. That is why one person is sensitive to gluten while another one may not be.

The bottom line is that the cause of the problem for any chronic health condition will be different for each patient and will remain unique to them. The aim is to find that root cause of your problem and treat it.

LEAKY GUT

I want to introduce you to the concept of "leaky gut" since it leads to many chronic and autoimmune diseases; it's one of the "root causes." Leaky Gut is a problem that occurs due to molecular mimicry which, if you remember, is when molecules copy or mimic each other, and a cross-reaction occurs because your immune system cannot distinguish between tissues, and unfortunately, antibodies are made against healthy and normal functioning glands, like the thyroid.

Our intestines have junctions that are tight. When we eat our food, it gets digested and absorbed in our intestines. These tight junctions can sometimes get leaky. This leak allows larger particles that don't usually make it through the intestine to pass. Thus, patients with leaky gut have toxins that get into their bloodstream, and from there, it causes an autoimmune reaction and inflammation that attacks the thyroid. You could then have symptoms of indigestion, including gas, bloating, and eructations, or you could experience cramping pain after eating a specific type of food.

Patients can end up living with all these symptoms for years and they haven't done anything about it, thinking that this is all just a part of life. But you don't have to feel this way. If you have any symptoms of leaky gut, have it checked. The way you absorb food and the way you feel may be completely different once this cause is addressed.

Causes of leaky gut are S.A.D. or the Standard American Diet, environmental toxins, sleep deprivation, alcohol, chronic stress, and liver toxicity. We must learn how to avoid these causes because without a healthy GI tract, it is impossible to have adequate defense against disease.

This picture explains the causes of leaky gut and how these toxins enter the blood-brain barrier and develop into an auto-immune disorder.

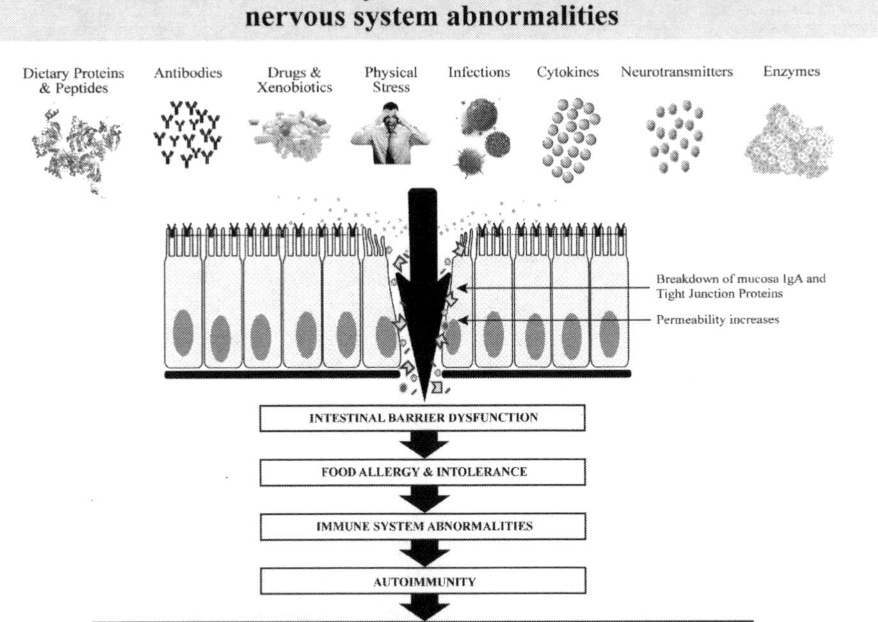
Factors affecting mucosal immune system resulting in intestinal barrier dysfunction, autoimmunity and nervous system abnormalities
Dietary Proteins & Peptides
Antibodies
Drugs & Xenobiotics
Physical Stress
Infections
Cytokines
Neurotransmitters
Enzymes
Breakdown of mucosa IgA and Tight Junction Proteins
Permeability increases
INTESTINAL BARRIER DYSFUNCTION
FOOD ALLERGY & INTOLERANCE
IMMUNE SYSTEM ABNORMALITIES
AUTOIMMUNITY
INFLUENCE ON THE BLOOD-BRAIN BARRIER AND NEUROAUTOIMMUNITY

FOOD SENSITIVITY TEST

A patient of mine with hypothyroidism and Hashimoto's thyroiditis was very frustrated. She was already on the right medication and supplements for her condition. She exercised regularly and followed the Paleo diet, which is kind of a caveman diet in which you only eat natural foods, much like our ancestors ate. She was an anxious type of person in general but regularly practiced stress management techniques like meditation. In spite of doing all of this, she was still having problems, such as weight gain, feeling fatigued, and poor sleep patterns.

I suggested for her to do a comprehensive food sensitivity test that tests for 154 foods. The test revealed that she was highly allergic to eggs, including the egg whites and egg yolk. And of course, since eggs are considered a great paleo food, she ate them all the time. Based on these test results, she eliminated eggs from her diet altogether.

I saw her again a month later and the difference was like night and day. She had high energy, no longer had digestive problems, was sleeping well, and felt like a new person overall. She felt like herself again. I re-tested her thyroid antibodies, and they dropped from somewhere in the 3000's to 300's in one month! Incredible. Removing eggs from her diet was the only change we had made in her treatment plan to help pinpoint the root cause of her problem. What this means is that, in her case, eggs were causing severe inflammation in her digestive tract, leading to her symptoms.

Yet, eggs are not harmful. The Paleo diet can be a healthy option for many people who want to lose weight. The problem is that not every person is the same.

I had a similar problem. Every morning, I would add spinach to my smoothie. You know spinach is considered a good food full of important minerals, including iron, which is vital for thyroid patients, as they can be iron deficient. Even the cartoon character Popeye the Sailorman agrees. For a snack, I would munch on almonds during the day, which are an excellent source of protein and healthy fats. Both spinach and almonds are considered health foods, but when I performed my own food sensitivity test, I found out that I reacted to them. After removing them from my diet for sometime, I saw an improvement in my symptoms.

Jeffrey Zavik, the founder of Immunolabs, says, "People never suspect that the reason they don't feel good, or the reason they can't lose weight, or they're depressed, or always feel tired, is actually because of the baked potato they had for lunch, or the corn in their soup, or the eggs they had for breakfast." Similarly, "Eating a green pepper may cause bloating and lethargy. Lemons may cause headaches. Still others could lose a few pounds if they removed eggs and soy from their diet. Without proper testing, these connections may go undetected."

A food sensitivity test will help you identify what is causing an inflammatory response rather than randomly removing the common allergens. But how do we find out this food sensitivity and allergic reaction?

This test is performed by a simple blood draw. Normally, the tests results come back within a week and show which foods your body is reactive and non-reactive to. You'll know which foods to avoid and which help your body's unique needs. It comes with a rotation diet plan for you to follow and you will have unlimited access to a Nutrition Expert who can help with recipes based on your results. It is a personalized approach. It's more than worth the cost.

Based on their test results, I ask my patients to completely avoid the foods they reacted to for 90 days and follow the rotation diet that's given to them. After that period, slowly introduce the foods that they reacted to, one at a time. If they don't have reactions to that food, they can re-introduce it back in their diet, but if they have a severe reaction, then they want to avoid it. For example, I had a patient who tested positive for wheat and thus avoided it for 90 days. She had excellent results, but when she re-introduced wheat after 90 days, she had severe cramping and vomiting, the worst reaction that she had experienced. Thus, she avoids wheat in her diet now and continues to do well.

You don't have to feel stressed about what to eat, as the labs have a nutrition expert that works with you. Also, don't feel that if you test positive on a particular food that you must avoid it for the rest of your life. That is generally not the case. Once you begin following a good rotation plan, you generally overcome those food sensitivities. The microbiome in your gut flourishes with the rotation diet.

Following the food sensitivity test plan has helped people of all ages. It could be a child with recurrent ear infections, a teenager diagnosed with ADD, a woman with mood disorders, someone diagnosed with IBS, or someone with chronic joint pains. If you are among those people who are having symptoms and have seen many doctors but found no help, then think "outside the box" and get yourself tested.

GI-MAP TEST

In the last few decades, DNA analysis has transformed the field of microbiology. The National Institutes of Health have followed suit with initiatives such as the Human Microbiome Project, which characterized the microbiome from over 15 habitats of the body in more than 200 healthy human subjects using DNA analysis. More than ever before, we are keenly aware of the health benefits or disease risks brought about by the microorganisms that inhabit the human body.

Culture techniques, previously the standard, left up to 50% of bacterial species virtually invisible. When next-generation methods revolutionized this field, it allowed the identification of tremendous numbers of previously unknown organisms. Anaerobic bacteria make up a large part of the human microbiome and can be opportunistic and cause illness. Therefore, inability to cultivate these organisms left a large blind spot for clinicians when trying to diagnose the source of infection.

The Gastrointestinal Microbial Assay Plus (GI-MAP) was designed to assess a patient's microbiome from a single stool sample, with particular attention to microbes that may be disturbing normal microbial balance and may contribute to perturbations in the gastrointestinal flora or illness. The panel is a comprehensive collection of microbial targets as well as immune and digestive markers. It screens for pathogenic bacteria, commensal bacteria, opportunistic pathogens, fungi, viruses, and parasites. It primarily uses automated DNA analysis to give practitioners a better view into the gastrointestinal microbiome.

The GI-MAP measures pathogenic organisms that can cause hospital-acquired infections (HAI) such as C. difficile or norovirus, foodborne illness such as E.coli or Salmonella, and common causes of diarrhea such as Campylobacter or Shigella. This panel measures viral causes of gastroenteritis, unavailable by other common stool tests. It measures parasites such as Cryptosporidium,

Giardia, and Entamoeba histolytica. The GI-MAP analyzes Helicobacter pylori and its virulence factors. It can detect opportunistic pathogens such as Pseudomonas aeruginosa, Klebsiella pneumoniae, and Proteus mirabilus, associated with autoimmune molecular mimicry. It includes a panel of single-celled, amoebic parasites such as Blastocystis hominis, Dientamoeba fragilis, and Entamoeba coli. Worms such as Necatur americanus and Trichuris trichuria are recent additions to the GI-MAP as well as cytomegalovirus and Epstein-Barr virus. Fungal organisms include Candida, Geotrichum, Microsporidia and more. Finally, the GI-MAP measures standard markers of immunity, inflammation, and digestion including calprotectin, secretory immunoglobulin A (sIgA), anti-gliadin antibody, and pancreatic elastase. Disruption of the gastrointestinal microbiome can cause GI symptoms like:

- Abdominal Pain
- Bloating
- Constipation
- Crohn's Disease
- Diarrhea
- Food Poisoning
- Gastric Cancer
- Gastritis
- Gastroenteritis

- Gastroesophageal Reflux
- Irritable Bowel Syndrome
- Small Intestinal Bacterial Overgrowth (SIBO) Gastrointestinal Symptoms
- Ulcerative Colitis
- Vomiting
- Autoimmune Conditions: Ankylosing Spondylitis, Reactive Arthritis, Rheumatoid Arthritis
- Allergic Disease: Asthma, Eczema. (Diagnostic Solutions Laboratory, 2017, p. 2)

I know the above was too much information. The point of it is that this type of comprehensive stool test looks for many more organisms that can be missed by a regular stool test by a conventional lab. It is a different type of analysis and is considered a functional test, the kind that Naturopathic and Integrative physicians like to run on their patients. It helps to find out what is causing the patient's GI symptoms. Is it SIBO, yeast, parasites, or is it leaky gut and inflammation? Or it may be a lack of digestive enzymes. It is beneficial to find the root cause of the problem so we can recommend appropriate treatment.

4-R'S TREATMENT APPROACH

I follow the 4 -R approach: Remove, Replace, Restore, and Repair.

REMOVE

Step one in the 4 -R approach is to Remove. Overgrowth of any pathogenic bacteria, yeast or parasites needs to be removed. Removal also refers to foods that are causing more harm to you than good.

SIBO - Small Intestinal Bacterial Overgrowth is starting to become a standard term. What it means is that there is an overgrowth of bacteria in the small intestine, a place where it should typically not be present. Oil of oregano, berberines, garlic, and olive leaf extract all have anti-microbial properties and will help against the bacterial overgrowth.

Candida and yeast infections - Overgrowth of yeast in the GI tract also causes many GI symptoms. I usually recommend a supplement with undecylenic acid, caprylic acid, and botanicals such as rosemary and thyme. They all create an action against yeast. I recommend the Candida diet, also called a Candida cleanse. Candida feeds on sugars, so this means a sugar-free diet for 90 days. It is also a yeast free diet, which means to avoid bread, wine, beer, and cheese. We're basically trying to starve the yeast.

Parasites - Usually a problem when you are traveling outside of the US. I like a tincture with sweet wormwood and black walnut. They both have a powerful action against parasites and can be used prophylactically when you travel.

In this section called "Remove," I would like to include the foods that should be removed from your diet.

An interesting and important side note is that if you have Hashimoto's, choosing to avoid gluten altogether could be a choice for you. Many who have eliminated it have seen improvements, including my patients. A study by Immunolabs found that when most of the people with subclinical hypothyroidism were placed on a gluten-free diet, their thyroid function normalized!

In 71% of people who strictly followed a one-year gluten withdrawal, there was a normalization of subclinical hypothyroidism. Another 19% of people who followed the gluten-free diet were able to normalize their thyroid antibodies. The researchers concluded, "In distinct cases, gluten withdrawal may single-handedly reverse the abnormality."

Yet not everyone who has a thyroid condition is sensitive to gluten. I'm not. This is where a food sensitivity test becomes essential. Every person is unique, and their reactions to food are different as well. A food sensitivity test will help you find out what specifically you are sensitive to and then remove those foods from your diet that are causing inflammation in your gut.

Remove processed foods from your life. It seems that people lack the understanding of food, including processed foods. So let me explain. Any food that looks different from its natural source is processed. Thus, everything that comes in a box or can is processed. When you walk into a grocery store, make sure that you shop for foods that are available in the fresh produce section and avoid the aisles in the middle of the store where you find processed foods.

People are not always familiar with the term "gluten." Gluten is present in wheat, rye, barley, and couscous. I once had a patient who said she was completely gluten-free. She avoided her cultural Indian bread called "Roti," which is made from whole wheat, but she ate all other kinds of bread, thinking that was gluten-free. Because of this, her diabetes was out of control.

An important thing is to not add extra sugars to your food. I treated a gentleman a couple of weeks ago and asked him how much soda he drank, thinking it would be a glass or two a day; he drank two liters of Dr. Pepper a day! Every day. I was in shock. Soda is filled with sugar and really should be avoided, especially in such amounts. Sugar, while delicious, is basically poison. It affects our hormones and cortisol levels, and as we eat it, we feel great, but then the sugar level drops, and we end up craving more. It's a vicious cycle.

Thus, you should avoid sugar when possible. Starbucks has a tempting section of desserts that you will notice when you go to pick up your coffee, but you should stay away from them. Also, avoid adding any sugar to your coffee or tea. It may taste bitter at first, but many times, people end up learning to enjoy the flavor without the extra sweetness.

Make life sweet, not your coffee.

REPLACE

Step two in the 4-R approach is to replace essential nutrients for proper utilization of food and facilitate digestion. Under Replace, I will also suggest a list of macronutrients (proteins, fats, and carbohydrates) that are good for you.

We can replace digestive enzymes, HCL, and bile salts if our body is under-producing any one or all of these. When we eat, our pancreas produces enzymes that help us to digest food. We must break down our carbohydrates, proteins, and fats. Your body must produce amylase, protease, and lipase to digest all three of those, but in some people, the pancreas does not produce enough of these enzymes to break down our foods. So what happens is if we don't make enough lipase and our fat doesn't get digested too well, one will notice undigested food particles in the stool. You wouldn't get the benefits of the healthy fat from the food you eat and, in turn, that affects your hormone production since hormones are made from cholesterol. Think about how everything is connected in our bodies, and if one part does not function optimally, it can affect many dependent functions. Thus, it is always important to find the root cause of the problem we are treating.

HCL is hydrochloric acid that is made in your stomach acid and is required for digesting proteins. Some people have low stomach acid and thus have a problem digesting proteins. Giving them Betaine HCl as a supplement will help this problem.

For example, when patients go through bariatric surgeries where they have gastric bypass or the stomach size is cut down so they don't feel as hungry, they're really compromising the functions of the stomach. Every part of our body has some important purpose, and if we remove one part of it, things get out of balance. If the stomach acid, HCl, is not there, we can't produce enough vitamin B12 or digest the protein. A lot of patients who come to see me after having these surgeries have symptoms of diarrhea or loose stools because they are unable to digest their foods adequately. They aren't absorbing nutrients from what they're eating since the food is going undigested. In the first place, they wanted to curb their appetite to get healthy, but they've compromised everything else. It's quite sad.

We must also replace all our unhealthy foods with healthy ones. But at this point, you may be wondering, especially since you haven't had a food sensitivity test yet, just what you can eat?

But first, before we get there, we need to correct some myths. These are foods you have been told you shouldn't eat, but you actually need.

Fat: Doesn't this word want to make you hop on a treadmill or relax into a yoga pose? But what if fat is a good thing, at least in your diet? The word "fat" has become such a terrifying thing that we don't even realize that we have cut out an essential part of nutrition. Saturated fats actually raise your good cholesterol (HDL).

I am a mother who breastfed her babies. Our bodies have the ability to heal themselves and milk adapts to what our newborns need; half of the fat in breastmilk is saturated fat. Saturated fat is so good for us because it cannot be oxidized. Saturated fats have a positive effect on our liver, hormones, and immunity. Yet it is best to stay away from saturated fats that come from processed foods. Instead, choose sources like coconut oil, organic butter, and ghee to cook your meals.

Another food curse word is cholesterol. You may think of a middle-aged man being told by his doctor that he must lower his cholesterol. He goes home to a breakfast of grapefruit instead of his beloved bacon, a frown on his face. You want to have a low LDL, yet our bodies need cholesterol. It is a vital part of cell membranes and is the starting substance from which your body makes all your hormones.

Carbs: The word that brought about a popular diet where we all were supposed to avoid bread and pasta. Yet we need plenty of carbohydrates. Carbs that help your body become healthy are colorful vegetables and fruits like berries, carrots, red bell peppers. Good carbs contain vitamins and minerals your body needs to function, to help you feel like yourself. Plus, they have fiber, which improves digestive function and nurtures your microbiome. People with hypothyroidism and Hashimoto's need to know that we need carbs to activate the T3 hormone. Remember that T3 is the one that our cells utilize to produce energy.

In general, eat a diet with a balance of macronutrients, which are proteins, good carbohydrates, and healthy fats. Make sure you choose the foods based on your food sensitivity test.

Here is a list of some good food sources for each macronutrient:

Proteins: eggs, fish, chicken, grass-fed meats, beans, lentils, yogurt, some dairy products, nuts, and seeds

Good carbs: vegetables, fruits, beans, and lentils, quinoa, steel-cut oats

Healthy fats: olive oil, coconut oil, nuts and seeds, avocados, and ghee

A simple tip to remember is if someone didn't

eat it 100 years ago, you shouldn't either. Avoid processed snack foods like those cheesy chips, don't drink your calories, and avoid all-purpose bleached flour, hydrogenated fats, and sugar, which is basically poison to humans.

There is a common saying, "We are what we eat." I would also add that we are what we digest and absorb. I believe this to be very true. We are made up of trillions of cells, and each cell requires nourishment to produce energy. If we provide them with good fuel in the form of food, we are going to be healthy.

Don't follow food trends; follow your body's needs.

RESTORE

Step three in the 4-R approach is where we must restore healthy bacteria in the gut. Probiotics restore healthy bacteria in your gut and can improve the production and regulation of key hormones like insulin, ghrelin, and leptin. They're even capable of raising immune function and protecting cognitive functioning. The best sources include yogurt, kefir, and cultured veggies, such as sauerkraut or kimchi, kombucha, and other fermented foods.

The GI Microbial Assay Plus (GI-MAP™) is very important to see which organisms are present in the gut, which will also help determine which probiotic will work best for you. Some people may require a prebiotic and others who may need a stronger one if they have had antibiotic-associated diarrhea.

Buying probiotics can become a little confusing, as there are thousands of strains available, but one that I particularly like is VSL #3. A standard probiotic has around 30 billion bacteria, which may sound great and is effective to a point. However, the VSL #3 has 112.5 billion bacteria per capsule and it needs to be refrigerated since the bacteria are live. This may seem like too much, but there are trillions of bacteria in our gut; thus, you do need a probiotic that has a good amount of live strains in it. I have used VSL #3 in my protocol for patients with Hashimoto's, and it has worked very well.

REPAIR

And finally, Step four in our 4-R approach would be to repair the gut. When the gut has been a habitat to unwanted bacteria, yeast, or parasites for a length of time, one develops inflammation and leaky gut from it. At that time, we need a protocol to heal and repair the gut. Botanicals that are mucilaginous like slippery elm, okra, aloe vera, and marshmallow have a healing effect on the gut. L-glutamine repairs the gut mucosa as well as supports the immune system. DGL (Deglycyrrhizinated Licorice) helps to repair gastric mucosa and also helps with symptoms of heartburn and bloating.

So, after sharing all this information, let me tell you that it all depends on synchrony. Like, if the pancreas is producing enough digestive enzymes to absorb the different foods that you are eating or does someone have an allergic reaction to foods that they are regularly consuming, or if there is an overgrowth of bacteria in the gut called SIBO, or do they have a yeast infection. All these things cause difficulty in digesting food. But we have tools to get to the root cause of the problem and help repair your gut.

WHICH DIET SHOULD I FOLLOW?

There are many popular diets out there right now, from the Paleo diet to Whole 30 and, while these may be good options for losing weight for some people, they don't always work for everyone.

Instead of focusing on a particular diet, we need to make sensible choices. Remember, we need to cut out processed foods. It seems easy, but even when products say non-GMO or gluten-free and are boxed or canned, it is not always great for you.

Here's a simple trick to stay away from processed foods. When you go to a grocery store, stick to the outside aisles that have fresh produce and foods and not the middle aisles where all the boxed, canned, and processed foods are. Another tip is that when you see food and it looks like where it came from, then the food is in its natural form.

I've had patients who think they are vegan, another popular diet. What they keep doing is eating everything soy from soy burgers to soy chips. Unfortunately, that's not healthy eating. It's made up food that's most likely processed. They could eat so many other healthy vegetarian proteins like lentils and beans.

People tend to think that a proper diet means eating no carbs, which is not good because we do need our carbs for energy. And for thyroid, the most active hormone, the T3 hormone, needs carbs to activate it. Good carbs are essential. If patients with hypothyroidism completely avoid carbs, they will be sluggish and run down.

It goes back to bio individualization. For example, with the Ketogenic diet, I will have one patient who loses weight and the other gain weight. That's why I have done my genetic test, to find out what diet suits me. For me, going on a high-fat diet like eating nut-butters and things like that means I'm just going to gain weight because my genetic panel showed that fat converts directly to fat for me. I do better with moderate carbs and protein as well. We can't generalize these diets; they have to be individualized. Having a genetic panel test can help you to find your unique dietary needs.

However, if you are unable to do this, there are a few foods I recommend my patients to eat.

Eat lean protein, a lot of vegetables, fruits, some healthy fats, and stay hydrated. With each meal, try to get some protein. For example, when you are snacking, you can have a little bit of cottage cheese with blueberries or an apple with almond butter. It helps not to eat the same food over and over. The more variety of healthy foods we have helps the microbiome and gut function.

You should eat about five or six times a day. Don't go hungry. I have patients who say they eat hardly anything but gain weight. Or they go the whole day without eating, then have a big meal in the evening. If you don't eat regularly, your metabolism slows down. Our bodies are smarter than we think. Eating these ways puts us into starvation mode because it's not getting food as fuel and will hold on to the weight and keep storing it as fat so it will have these reserves for later.

What you don't want to do is to cut something out forever. If you see a piece of cake once in a while, take a little bit. Have a couple bites so you can feel like you enjoyed it. You don't have to have big pieces, but these small amounts will make you feel like you're not depriving yourself of anything. You can have your treats occasionally but eat the healthy choices all the time.

Really, the best thing I have found to help you lose weight is to realize there isn't a perfect diet; eat five to six times a day using the foods mentioned above, drink water, and have a moderate amount of exercise. Think moderation and sensible.

GENETIC TESTING

"Losing and maintaining weight has never seemed harder for many patients. The extra pounds contribute to a myriad of health issues and can also result in a destructive cycle of shame and self-blame, which impedes the healing process further. With an array of potential diet plans now available, it can be a challenge to know which approach to recommend for each patient, especially considering that one diet may work for your friend but not for you. Each person is unique. Thankfully, the Kashi Weight Management Panel takes the guesswork out of determining the right plan by going straight to genetics for the answers" (Kashi Labs, n.d., para. 1).

Over a decade ago, a major evolution took place in the field of technology. In the mid-90s, I remember learning the MS-DOS as an operating system for personal computers. My first computer project was using a floppy disk. Times rapidly changed, and we went from floppy disks as data storage to CDs, hard drives, jump drives, and what not. After a while, I was unable to keep up, since I am not a tech savvy person to begin with. I knew that there was a huge change that happened in the computer world, and soon enough with the world wide web, people could have their own websites and share their information with the world with great ease. I bring this to your attention since I think that the field of Genomics is at that stage now where it will be readily accessible to the world.

My husband, Apurva Patel, has worked for TGEN (Translational Genomics Research Institute) for a decade. He always told me that knowing genome sequencing is the way to personalized medicine, and ten years later, I see it for real.

Genome sequencing started as a very complex and an expensive affair. Only a handful of people were able to afford it then. 23andME began a genetic service that was available for people to access, understand, and benefit from the human genome. A couple years ago, few patients had ordered this test for themselves and brought in the data to share with me. At that time, the reports looked complex, and I did not know what to do with it. Also, initially, people thought that by analyzing their genes, they were going to find out how they were going to die. This reason would not interest people like me to do this kind of a test. I am interested in this type of testing now because I am finding a new twist to it. With the interpretation of the genetic test, one can find out what steps they can take to promote health and wellness. It is always easy to align with the positive information rather than the negative. People would rather know how they can live a good healthy life rather than know how they will die, by interpreting their genes!

Many labs have emerged that are providing a wide variety of genetic panels. These include cardiac health panel, bone health panel, behavioral health panel, etc. You may either choose to order a comprehensive panel encompassing many different genetic tests and markers or decide to request a specific panel that you are interested in. I tried out the weight management panel for myself, and the results were spot on. I did this panel through Kashi labs. It was effortless. I had to send in three buccal swabs, which took less than two minutes to swab/collect and package. The results elaborated the gene markers tested for, and based on the results, recommended food intake goals for fats, proteins, and carbohydrates, and recommended exercise intensity.

The Kashi Weight Management Panel determines the right plan for you by going straight to genetics for the answers. Their test provides analysis of genes highly associated with weight gain and elevated body mass index (BMI). Using your results, they offer dietary and lifestyle recommendations that are scientifically supported to help get the fastest results without all the trial-and-error of dieting. For many, a personalized weight management strategy tailored to their genetic code can make a significant impact. It may make an impact for you as well and is something to consider.

Weight Management Panel

Kashi Clinical Laboratories has a useful panel for weight management on their site that you can find here:

Genetic Markers Included in the Weight Management Panel	
TEST CATEGORIES	EFFECTS ON NUTRITIONAL HEALTH
FTO	Appetite Regulation, Calorie Intake, Frequent Cravings
MC4R	Appetite Regulation, Carbohydrate Digestion, Metabolism Regulation, Insulin Regulation
FABP2	Dietary Fat Sources, Fat Utilization, Metabolism Regulation, Insulin Regulation
ADRB2	Physical Activity, Carbohydrate Digestion, Insulin Regulation
SH2B1	Leptin Production, Carbohydrate Cravings, Insulin Regulation

Ideal Candidates are Patients with the Following Symptoms or Conditions:

- Poor Results from Prior Dietary Changes
- Frequent Cravings and Over-eating
- Sedentary Lifestyle
- Persistent Weight Gain
- High BMI (>25)
- Weight Gain in The Stomach, Hips, and Thighs.

The above is just a snip of the vast information our genes can provide. I recently watched Dr. Yael Joffe, Rd, Ph.D.'s video on Interpretation of a Genetic Test. She went into the details of the DNA life testing. It was excellent information, and I became interested in testing myself. The impact of diet, lifestyle, exercise, and environment on an individual's genetic makeup should not be underestimated. "Knowledge of how external factors influence genes enables the development of personalized health programs not only in supporting the chronically ill patient to improve health but also for someone at peak fitness levels to gain the most from their training program" (DNA Life, 2018, para. 3).

I recently hosted Dr. Christina Tondora on my talk show on Facebook, and her topic was Your DNA is NOT your Destiny. She talked about how easy it is to do the DNA test that she offers to her patients, and it is only a one-time test that provides a wealth of information personalized for you so that you can make the right choices in your life.

"There is an emerging revolution in healthcare that will lead to a kind of medicine with new dimensions-it will be predictive, preventive, personalized and participatory- P4 medicine."

- Lee Hood, MD, PhD

Using these methods, eating not just healthy, but the right foods for your body's individual needs, will help you improve your gut, thyroid, and overall health. You can feel like yourself once more. What you eat is your choice. Your gut health depends on you to make the right choices, and a doctor like me can lead you in the right direction.

WHERE TO START?

Your health starts with the gut, so start with what you eat. Since it may take some time before you can have a food sensitivity test, you can begin by removing common allergens, such as dairy, corn, soy, eggs, sugar, and especially gluten, as a high number of patients are sensitive to gluten. Avoid processed and fried foods as well (sorry, ranch-flavored chips) by staying in the outside aisles in your grocery store, where you will find fresh produce and foods. Perform the food sensitivity test to find out what foods may be causing allergic reactions in your gut; it could even be something healthy that you are eating routinely like almonds and spinach. And please refer to the list of Thyroid Healing Foods.

Having healthy bacteria in your gut is essential. Flourish your microbiome by rotating your foods. If you are having digestive problems, consider the GI Map test to rule out the underlying cause of the problem so that it can be eliminated. It will even test for leaky gut, inflammation, and gluten sensitivity.

If you want to find out which diet will work best for you, ask your genes! Following a genetic-based test yields good results rather than guessing which diet to follow, since so many are available. You will not only lose weight but heal your thyroid and feel like yourself again.

STEP 4:

REDUCE TOXIC ENVIRONMENTAL EXPOSURE

By age ten, a child born in 2000 is exposed to approximately 80,000 chemicals that did not exist in 1970.

When I lived in India, we had pest control people come every three months to spray chemicals in our yard that killed the bugs. Their huge tube-like machine exhaled some toxic fumes that caused a gassy haze. As kids, we were fascinated by this cloud of gas since we could get lost in the smog. At that time, nobody stopped us. Nobody thought anything of it. One time after playing in that smog, I was sick for three days with a high fever. It was so toxic. These chemical toxins really messed me up and may have contributed to my Hashimoto's later in life.

Environment, especially heavy metals, play an important role in the health of your thyroid. We must know about metal toxicity because of the influence it has on the thyroid. These heavy metals directly latch on to the thyroid and lower its functioning as it affects the conversion of the T4 to the active T3 hormone.

Common Heavy Metals

The common heavy metals are mercury, lead, cadmium, and arsenic.

Mercury is a neurotoxin that comes from fish that we eat and dental amalgams. In high doses, it can kill a person, but in small amounts, it affects your nervous system and heart. If you are living with these fillings, then you have a mercury toxicity exposure all the time. The good news is these days you can find a holistic or natural dentist that can help you have the fillings replaced with a nontoxic material.

Personally, I'm not a seafood eater, but this is good for you to know. Fish also contain mercury, especially larger fish. Fish like tuna, tilefish, king mackerel, swordfish, and shark will carry more and more mercury from the smaller fish they eat. Look for smaller fish, such as salmon or tilapia, which may contain lower levels of mercury. When you buy fish oils, look for mercury-free oils. Nordic Naturals is a good brand. The symptoms of mercury toxicity are insomnia, anxiety, and possibly cancer.

Lead affects many organs in your body and has a variety of health effects, ranging from hearing loss and nervous system problems to permanent brain damage. People who are close to or over 40 have been exposed to lead growing up. It comes from paint in houses and from lead pipes that carried drinking water. Lead will store in your bones and on the thyroid tissue, diminishing thyroid function and lowering thyroid hormone production.

Arsenic is also a well-known toxin. You may have read a murder mystery story where a woman kills someone by poisoning them with arsenic, but arsenic is found in natural places like water. In places where someone uses well water, arsenic will be prevalent. While you're not likely to find mercury or lead in your water at home, you may find arsenic and be poisoning yourself without even knowing it. It's a good idea to get a filter. Doses found in water can cause different kinds of cancers, birth defects, and more.

The last chemical is cadmium, which is found with cigarette smoke and car exhaust, which is also important to avoid, just as I should have avoided or been told to stay away from the smog in my childhood. Cadmium may cause breathing problems and kidney damage as well as cancers.

The toxicity from these heavy metals and toxins deplete and affect your energy levels because they affect your powerhouse, the mitochondria. So, if they are affected, not just the energy you feel but the kind that keeps your body running will be really low.

Mitochondria take in the nutrients, break them down, and create energy-rich molecules for the cell. An average human body contains approximately 37.2 trillion cells! So think about how many cells we need to provide nutrients to produce energy. What occurs when mitochondria get stressed? Apoptosis, which means the death of the cells. This will lead to end-organ diseases. Please see the table to understand which body systems are affected and what are the early and late stage diseases that can occur due to mitochondria damage.

BODY SYSTEMS	EARLY EFFECTS	END ORGAN DISEASES
Immune System	Frequent infections Chronic inflammation	Life-threatening infections (Pneumonia, MRSA, etc.)
Hepatic System	Elevated Liver function tests Chemical sensitivities	NASH, Hepatitis, Cancer
Nervous System	Decreased cognition Brain fog, fatigue	Alzheimer's dz, MS, ALS, Parkinson's dz, Chronic Fatigue Syndrome

How do we support healthy mitochondrial function so it can produce sustained energy?

1. **Healthy Food Intake** - "We are what we eat" is a popular saying, but it is 100% true. If we have clean eating habits, we will not only have more energy but prevent long-term chronic and degenerative diseases. While if we have unclean eating habits, we will feel tired and lethargic and will cause inflammation in our gut, leading to chronic diseases.

   What does clean eating include? Vegetables, fruits, nuts/seeds, ancient grains, healthy fats, and lean protein. Besides making healthy food choices, the times that the food is consumed also matters. Fasting for a day a week or intermittent fasting helps utilize fat as fuel and helps you feel more energetic and have a clearer mind.

2. **Mitonutrient Therapy** - Optimal levels of all the micronutrients is essential for the healthy functioning of mitochondria. I like to run the micronutrient test on my patients because it checks for all the vitamins, minerals, and antioxidant levels, and provides a comprehensive ten-page report that helps me personalize treatments for my patients by finding which nutrients they are specifically deficient in at an intracellular level. Did you know that being on certain common prescription medications depletes nutrients

and thus leads to mitochondrial damage?

A key triad of mitochondrial support ingredients are:

- **Acetyl L-Carnitine** - directly works on the mitochondria and helps the brain work better. It promotes biosynthesis of acetylcholine, a key neurotransmitter for brain and nerve function. In clinical studies, it has shown to benefit cognitive ability, memory, and mood.

- **N-acetyl Cysteine** - is a readily available, inexpensive amino acid derivative. It plays a role in restoring intracellular levels of the body's most powerful antioxidant, glutathione. It is effective against a constellation of chronic degenerative diseases, including impaired glucose control and cancer.

- **Alpha Lipoic Acid** - is an antioxidant and high doses of it have been used in parts of Europe for certain types of nerve damage. Studies suggest that it helps with type 2 diabetes. Studies show that it might help with dementia and some other studies suggest that as a cream, it might help skin damage related to aging.

3. **Movement Activities** - we know that it is important to exercise. Many times, the excuse is that "I can't find time during the day to exercise." Yes, I agree. It can sound like an excuse, but for many, it's not. I am in the same boat. Working full-time and raising two kids keeps me occupied enough. Even though I would love to join a class or go to the gym, I don't have the time for that.

   So, what are some alternatives?

   - Do a ten-minute exercise video watching YouTube.

   - Do 50 jumping jacks, three times a day, in the morning before work, during lunch break, and then in the evening. There are benefits to short-term high-intensity exercise. It will boost your metabolism and keep energy levels high.

4. **Stress Reduction** - My mantra this year has been that I will not do anything that causes stress in my life. It has given me a chance to focus on doing that nourishes my soul. In the process, I am learning not to care about what people think of me, stay away from small talk, which I never enjoyed, and stay focused on my path. I focused my energy towards writing my first book, which you are reading right now. Stress is linked to so many chronic diseases and is not worth it. Life is too short, and we don't know what

it will bring tomorrow, so we might as well enjoy everything we do.

5. **Spiritual Practice** - This is a must. Something that connects you to your true self. I have been working on this by meditation, reading books, and listening to inspirational authors. If you can't do it by yourself, then join a group. It could mean being a part of a church and going there every Sunday and getting involved in community activities. Serving others brings utmost satisfaction to the heart.

The above information about the Mitonutrient Therapy is by Dr. Jon Kaiser, who is a founder of K-Pax Pharmaceuticals. He has been treating patients with Chronic Fatigue Syndrome, HIV/AIDS, cancer, and other immune system disorders for the past twenty-five years. He has developed formulas to support mitochondria called Mitonutrients, which are made by Integrative Therapeutics. Please refer to this website to read published articles in Mitochondrial Medicine.

www.hopeforfatigue.org

PLASTIC CONTAINERS - PHTHALATES EXPOSURE

We now live longer than any other time in history. We have modern science and medicine that is curing diseases. We are advanced, and yet, we are poisoning ourselves for the future. One way in which we are doing this is through the phthalates and plastics in our food.

It is practically impossible to live without being exposed to heavy metals or toxins since they are present everywhere. A few thyroid toxins are BPAs, fluoride, and triclosan. Triclosan is in our antibacterial soaps and phthalates are present in many places, like our fragrances and plastic.

How easy is it to pop a little meal in the microwave that promises to make you lean and smiling? It has greens, veggies, and protein with only a few calories. Thus, it sounds like a perfect health solution. But yet again, this is a point where it's tricky to avoid toxins.

This time, the danger is in the plastic container that the food sits on. The soft, flexible plastic may contain phthalates, which can cause a wide range of health problems, including damage to your lungs, kidneys, and liver as well as cause thyroid abnormalities. We may only absorb a small amount of phthalates, but over a period of time, they become harmful. When plastic is heated, it leaches more of the chemicals, so keep your containers out of the dishwasher or microwave. Glass is a safer option when avoiding toxins.

PESTICIDE USE IN FOOD

Pesticides are also found in the food you buy, such as produce, meat, and dairy. Go certified organic since the use of pesticides is not allowed, and once again, avoid processed foods. The trick I mentioned in Step 3 applies here too; if a person didn't eat a certain food 100 years ago, you shouldn't either.

Pesticides have become prevalent for farmers, as they are a way to grow crops. Yet these pesticides can be leftover on the food you buy. Therefore, it is better to buy certified organic to avoid any of the remnants, as pesticides can play a role in disrupting your hormones and thus, your thyroid.

EWG- Dirty Dozen & Clean 15

Thinking about how hard it is to avoid toxins and heavy metals in your environment can make you wonder what you can put on the dinner table that'll be safe for you and your family. The Environmental Working Group's Shopper's Guide to Pesticides identifies fruits and vegetables that have the highest and lowest pesticide residues. These 15 fruits and vegetables, which make up their "Clean 15" list, are least likely to be contaminated with pesticide residues. They have what they call

Clean 15, foods that are generally safe to eat that are not organic.

EWG also put out a great list on the opposite spectrum called The Dirty Dozen, foods you should always buy organic as they may contain pesticides or, in other words, dirty.

CLEAN 15	**DIRTY DOZEN**
Sweet Corn	Strawberries
Avocados	Spinach
Pineapples	Nectarines
Cabbage	Apples
Onions	Peaches
Frozen Sweet Peas	Pears
Papayas	Cherries
Asparagus	Grapes
Mangos	Celery
Eggplant	Tomatoes
Honeydew	Sweet Bell Peppers
Kiwi	Potatoes
Cantaloupe	
Cauliflower	
Grapefruit	

I encourage you to explore more topics and stay updated with lists at www.ewg.org. This is the best source to look for when you are making choices about food, skin care products to choose from, etc.

TESTING AND TREATMENTS FOR HEAVY METAL EXPOSURE

What if you have already been exposed? The likelihood is high, but heavy metals can be removed from your body.

When I went to medical school, we learned about chelation. This is a method where, depending on the kind of heavy metal found, we'd find the best binding substance to bind to the heavy metal and then remove it from one's body. First, the patient was checked for heavy metal toxic exposure by a urine test, and then, based on those results, a chelating substance was chosen to remove the metal from the body. Chelation can be done by a weekly IV or using an oral chelating agent. We rechecked the levels after a matter of weeks to see how they were improving with the treatment. While undergoing treatment, they may have experienced symptoms as if going through a detox, such as headaches, brain fogginess, or nausea.

But now the current treatment focuses on the liver cleansing. I like what Dr. Shade has been working on, where he uses the mercury tri-test. The tri-test will help determine where the source of mercury is from. For example, if it's inorganic mercury, we know then that it's coming from the dental amalgams, and if its organic mercury, it's coming from fish. This way, we can tell a patient what they need to work on and how to remove or stop the mercury toxin exposure. Maybe they will need to have their dental treatment redone or look for fish without mercury.

Detoxification of the Liver

It is important that we treat the liver, since its job is to remove toxins from the body. We need to get rid of some of the toxins that have built up over time in the liver, and we can do this using herbs like milk thistle, intravenous glutathione, N-Acetyl-Cysteine (glutathione precursor), and Vitamin C. Make organic food choices as much as possible and eat veggies and fruits, or plant-based foods.

There are so many types of cleanses out there, but what we are trying to do is to get rid of all the bad foods and support the liver, so that it's working well to process everything. The liver, over the long term, is affected the most since it is processing all kinds of food and environmental toxins. This is why I recommend a ten-day supervised Naturopathic Cleanse.

A few symptoms that could indicate you need a cleanse would be fatigue, brain fogginess, and irritability.

This cleanse is best done twice a year during the spring and fall. You can think of it as a holiday or vacation for your body. While on the cleanse, there are certain foods that you will mostly eat, like vegetables and fruits. Fresh juice is a great option. We also use some liver supporting herbs, like milk thistle, glutathione, and even a mild laxative to keep your bowels going and flushing all the toxins from your body. With a healthy detox, you will have higher energy, since your body isn't working so hard to process and remove all the bad foods. Your mood will be better, as well as your energy. I've seen patients lose up to five pounds on a detox.

This may even be a good time to do a mental detox. Mental detox includes taking a break from electronics, phone, and thus from constant stimulation. It's a time to look inward. Practice meditation, journaling, having your daily golden hour, or taking a walk through nature. Doing this mental and physical detox will give you and your body a much-needed break.

Glutathione

One way to treat any toxicity is to support your liver with nutrients and herbs. The liver is the natural filter for your body, cleaning out all the toxins, so if it works well, it can help excrete some of the thousands of chemicals and heavy metal toxins we encounter on a day-to-day basis.

Dr. Joe Pizzorno mentions glutathione and the three ways it is important in the Broken Brain Series:

Glutathione is the most important antioxidant, and it helps with the detoxification. We want to stimulate anything that upregulates the glutathione, as it does three things that are vital to your health.

1. Glutathione predicts how long a species lives based on its ability to produce it. This is because it is the most important antioxidant in your body and in your mitochondria. If your levels are low, your DNA, cells, and mitochondria will degenerate more quickly.

2. It helps your liver get rid of chemicals from your body.

3. Glutathione is responsible for excreting mercury out of your brain through the blood-brain barrier, plus it aids in getting mercury out of your cells.

Glutathione is a well-kept secret weapon of your body, one that will have you losing the battle to a healthy thyroid without.

There are a few ways you can boost your glutathione: intravenously or orally from supplements that are high in broccoli extracts. Broccoli sprouts are the largest inducers of glutathione production.

"Consume sulfur-rich foods. The main ones in the diet are garlic, onions, and the cruciferous vegetables (broccoli, kale, collards, cabbage, cauliflower, watercress, etc.)" (Martino, 2017, para. 6). Try bioactive whey protein. This is a great source of cysteine and the amino acid building blocks for glutathione synthesis.

WHERE TO START?

Take a look once more at the Clean 15 and Dirty Dozen. If you have your house sprayed for bugs, don't let your children play around that area or stop altogether. You don't want you or your children to wind up with a fever for days, or possibly with Hashimoto's like I did when I followed behind the smog from the pest control contraption. Get a filter for your faucet water. Try to go green, not only with food but with makeup and fragrances as well. And last, try not use plastic containers, as they may contain phthalates. If that seems impossible, try not heating them in the microwave and wash by hand.

Do a Naturopathic Cleanse for ten days every spring and fall. Your liver needs time to detoxify for all the work it does for you throughout the year.

Removing these toxins and heavy metal is another way to elevate your energy levels by giving your mitochondria a boost and make your thyroid work better so you don't have to push yourself every day to accomplish tasks. You'll feel more like yourself again.

Change is the only constant. Stay on top of things and be resilient. I love being part of a medical community that has an open mind and who want to help people with the best treatments available that Do No Harm (one of the six principles of Naturopathic Medicine).

STEP 5: BALANCE YOUR HORMONES

Growing up in India, I watched my grandmother go through menopause. She would have a tough time falling asleep at night (it was considered "normal" for her to get three hours of sleep at night), so she watched TV instead. As kids, we used to love doing up her hair, and we needed many hairpins to hold her bun. Over the years, I saw her lose her hair and, again, it was considered as part of "aging." On the other hand, my maternal grandmother went through multiple mood changes and was diagnosed with severe depression—she had to go through rounds of harsh electroconvulsive therapy, where a brain seizure is induced to lift the person from depression.

It was hard to see a loved one go through a time like this. I wish someone would have known how to help her, as I help women now. It is my passion to help women feel their best at every stage of life, and to do this, we have to make sure that her hormones are balanced and working in harmony.

All the hormones in your body work in synchrony. The thyroid is your gland for metabolism, the adrenal glands control your stress response and sit on top of your kidneys, and the pituitary gland lies under your brain and is the master gland. It sends signals to other glands and regulates the hormones produced by these glands. The pituitary gland sends signals to the thyroid in the form of TSH like we've talked about, to the ovarian gland (FSH and LH), and to the adrenal glands (ACTH). Notice how all the pituitary signals end in H.

The pituitary gland controls the hormone production by sending signals through a negative feedback loop. That means, when TSH levels increase, that the thyroid is not functioning optimally and is under-producing thyroid hormones. When FSH levels increase, it means the ovaries are not producing enough estrogen, which tells me that a woman is in perimenopause, leading towards menopause. All these hormones made by different glands work in synchrony. So, if there is one gland that is not working well, the other gland can pick up the slack and work harder to compensate for the one that is under-producing. It can do this to some extent. For example, when thyroid production is low, the adrenal glands work harder to support the thyroid. But beyond a point, they will not be able to continue supporting, and thyroid treatment may be required.

The ovaries produce the female sex hormones, estrogen, progesterone, and testosterone.

When I see a patient for hormone balancing, I like to run all hormone tests at the initial consult so I get the whole picture. It consists of checking a complete thyroid panel, adrenal panel, and a female sex hormone panel. For the adrenal panel, I check the AM cortisol levels and the DHEA-S. While for female sex hormones, I check estradiol, progesterone, testosterone, and FSH (follicle stimulating hormone).

I like to see the whole picture, but if I see a hormonal imbalance in more than one panel, I will begin by correcting one hormonal imbalance at a time. If I started with correcting all three imbalances, I would not know which treatment is helping my patient. If I have already balanced your estrogen, progesterone, and testosterone levels to help with you with perimenopause and menopause, yet you're still suffering from symptoms of low energy and slow metabolism, I would then run a complete thyroid panel. Once the thyroid is corrected, patients feel like themselves again. They've lost weight, have more energy, and generally feel better.

When I explain the hormone results to women, some of them break down in tears saying how they have talked about this with their doctor for 10-15 years and nothing was offered to help them. They were struggling and pushing through from day to day just like I had, but now they finally had an answer.

Hormones During Various Stages in a Woman's Life

Women's hormones fluctuate and change most during these three stages of life: Puberty, Pregnancy and Lactation, and Menopause. Thyroid disorders are usually diagnosed when a woman is in one of these stages.

Hormones influence a young girl's life starting in puberty. A balance of hormonal rhythms will regulate her natural menstrual cycles. Her body needs to make sufficient hormones to support a healthy pregnancy. There comes a time when the ovaries stop producing adequate hormones, and she goes from peri-menopause to menopause. The lack of these hormones brings along a long list of symptoms, which may vary from person to person.

In the mid-thirties, the testosterone levels begin to drop when a woman notices that she may quickly get tired, notices more fat on her body and decline of muscle mass, has low libido and anxiety. Her memory seems to decline. For example, she forgets names or dates that she remembered before or forgets where she kept her keys. She begins to lose interest in sex and may have mood swings or anxiety.

Then, as she reaches closer to menopause, estrogen and progesterone levels decline, which brings on menopause and its classic symptoms of hot flashes, night sweats, mood swings, sleep problems, and pain during sex due to vaginal dryness. Besides the above symptoms, post-menopause is the time when she is at increased risk of developing chronic diseases like osteoporosis, cardiovascular disease, diabetes, breast, and colon cancer.

MENOPAUSE

Menopause is a time in a woman's life when her hormones begin to change significantly. It is often a time when thyroid disorders are diagnosed. The three stages of menopause are peri-menopause, menopause, and post-menopause.

1. Perimenopause is when you are getting close to menopause and your hormone levels begin to fluctuate and is usually the beginning of symptoms of menopause.

2. Menopause is when your ovaries stop producing the sex hormones, bringing a pause to your menstrual cycles.

3. Post-menopause is all the years after menopause.

But how do you know when you are in menopause?

The standard way of diagnosing it was that a woman does not have any menstrual bleeding for one year, yet every woman goes through menopause differently. For some women, their periods may stop one day and never come back. For others, their menstrual cycles may get farther apart. They may go two or three months between the bleeding period, whereas others may have cycles that start coming closer together. The bleeding amounts can vary, increase, or decrease. They may have more clots with bleeding. The symptoms are unique to each woman.

You can also look for any of the following symptoms:

1. **Hot flashes or night sweats:** can present in different ways. Some women experience it in the form of flushing that comes and goes, and others may feel hot all the time. Some women wake up in the middle of the night drenched in sweat.

2. **Sleep problems:** Some women have difficulty falling asleep while others can fall asleep but will wake up in the middle of the night, unable to fall back asleep.

3. **Weight gain:** As the female hormones decline during menopause, women find it difficult to lose weight or may gain weight. They feel flabby with lack of muscle tone.

The body fat percentage increases.

4. **Mood Swings:** Moods can fluctuate from depression to anxiety. One may feel down and cry very easily. These women come and tell me that they never used to be like this before. Once a Type A woman, she has now transitioned into a dull, sulky person who lacks the motivation to get even small things done.

5. **Brain Fog:** Notice difficulty in remembering things. May stop in the middle of the sentence because she lost the train of her thought. Puts the key somewhere and looks for it everywhere! Previously a super mom and multi-tasking, now finds it difficult to get one thing done.

6. **Dryness:** The texture of the skin and hair begins to change. The wrinkles start to appear as the skin gets dry. She may even experience hair loss. Her natural lubrication declines; thus a woman experiences vaginal dryness and painful intercourse. The joints begin to ache due to lack of lubrication between the joints.

It is a difficult and uncomfortable time for many women and something we must all go through to live a long life. Yet, there are ways to help a woman transition through menopause, smoothly and naturally.

1. Testing

First and foremost is to find out if a woman is in menopause. Bloodwork can be ordered using a regular lab, which includes FSH and Estradiol levels. When FSH (Follicle Stimulating Hormone) consistently tests 20 or more, it tells me that a woman is in menopause. Estradiol levels, which usually fluctuate during the menstrual cycles, begin testing consistently low during and post-menopause.

Nowadays, there are more advanced labs available that look at the breakdown of estrogen and its metabolites, which helps to find out if the body is making a good or bad kind of estrogen. Genetic testing can be combined to find out the risk of breast cancer if a woman has a family history of it.

2. Treatment

Botanical Medicine

Many women are determined to utilize therapies that are herbal or nutritional or combined with natural hormones to create a risk-to-benefit ratio that they feel comfortable with.

Red Clover — At least four clinical trials have been conducted on the effect of red clover isoflavones on vasomotor symptoms. Two show benefit and two do not. The first two published studies on red clover and vasomotor symptoms showed no statistically significant difference between the red clover standardized extract and the placebo during a three-month period, although both groups did improve. Two other studies of 40 mg standardized extract of red clover produced a reduction in hot flushes and night sweats. The most recent study showed that 80 mg of red clover isoflavones per day reduced the frequency of hot flashes by 44%.

Black Cohosh — Black cohosh has emerged as the single most important herb for the treatment of menopausal symptoms. There have been six well-publicized studies. In one of the most extensive studies, 629 women with menopausal complaints were given a standardized liquid extract of black cohosh twice per day for six to eight weeks.

As early as four weeks, 80 percent of women saw clear improvements in their menopausal ailments. Complete disappearance of symptoms occurred in approximately 50 percent. Symptoms included hot flashes, night sweats, headaches, insomnia, and mood swings. The other studies reported improvements in fatigue, irritability, hot flashes, and vaginal dryness.

Ginseng — Panax ginseng, also known as Korean or Chinese ginseng, contains at least 13 different triterpenoid saponins, collectively known as ginsenosides. Whether it involves reducing mental or physical fatigue, enhancing the ability to cope with various physical and mental stressors by supporting the adrenal glands, or treating the atrophic vaginal changes due to lack of estrogen, ginseng is a valuable tool for many menopausal women.

Homeopathic medicine

Here is a list of five homeopathic remedies commonly prescribed for hot flashes:

Lachesis — The person needing this homeopathic remedy typically experiences flushes of heat primarily on falling asleep, through the night, or on waking.

Sulphur — The woman needing this homeopathic remedy often feels warm and is worse from heat. The hot flashes tend to ascend the body, rising to the face and head, which may often feel hot. They may also frequently experience being too hot at night in sleep, especially the feet, which they desire to uncover.

Sepia — A person needing this homeopathic remedy often has hot flashes that are typically accompanied by weakness, lots of sweating, with the feeling of heat usually ascending upwards. Sepia patients typically are better from hard workouts or exertion and can be emotionally sensitive and a bit nervous by nature.

Pulsatilla — This remedy would be most often indicated in a menopausal woman who has become very sensitive, down, blue, and weepy. She feels better from reassurance. The hot flashes are worse in a warm room and better outside in cold or fresh air.

Glonoinum — A woman needing this homeopathic remedy often has hot flushes that are sudden, violent, and with an upward rush of blood to the head. Palpitations in the chest are also common, as are bursting headaches rising up from the neck, with great throbbing and sense of expansion as if the head would burst.

Diet

When trying to balance hormones and reduce menopause symptoms, your diet should include plenty of essential minerals and healthy fats. Filling up on the following foods which are "hormone-balancing," nutrient-dense, and unprocessed can help you eliminate your intake of empty calories and manage weight gain.

Organic fruits and vegetables — These contain dietary fiber to manage your appetite, antioxidants to slow the aging process, and phytosterols that can help balance hormones.

Cruciferous vegetables — Vegetables in the cruciferous family, such as broccoli, cabbage, and kale, contain indole-3-carbinol, which naturally helps to balance estrogen levels, although you want to avoid excess consumption of them since they are considered goitrogens and can affect thyroid adversely.

Healthy fats and cold-pressed oils — It's true that fats have more calories than protein or carbohydrates do, but they are also the building blocks for hormone production, keep inflammation levels low, boost your metabolism, and promote satiety, which is important for preventing weight gain. Unrefined oils provide essential vitamin E that helps regulate estrogen production. Look for virgin coconut oil, palm oil, extra-virgin olive oil, and flaxseed oil. Other sources of healthy fats include avocado, coconut milk, nuts, seeds, and wild seafood.

Probiotic foods — Probiotics are healthy bacteria that can improve your production and regulation of key hormones like insulin, ghrelin, and leptin. They're even capable of raising immune function and protecting cognitive functioning. The best sources include yogurt, kefir, cultured veggies such as sauerkraut or kimchi, kombucha, and other fermented foods.

Essential oils — Clary sage oil is the most effective essential oils for balancing hormones. It can help offer relief from menopause symptoms, including increased anxiety and hot flashes. In addition, roman chamomile oil reduces stress, peppermint oil can help cool the body from hot flashes, and thyme oil can help naturally balance hormones.

Have you thought about this, that all these chronic diseases like osteoporosis, heart disease, hypertension, and cancer can have an association with the drop in your hormone levels? Yes, it is true. What can we do to prevent these diseases and help get rid of all the symptoms that are impacting life in a huge way? Not only does the woman suffer by herself, but her family suffers too because of what she is going through, primarily due to her fluctuating moods.

My practice tends to focus more on women, yet women are not the only ones who go through hormonal changes. Men don't have an obvious cycle like women do, so they can't tell when they go through these changes. Andropause sounds like menopause! Men become cranky, lazy, gain weight around the mid-abdomen, and their libido drops.

Men are hormonal as well.

Bioidentical Hormone Replacement Therapy

After my graduation as a Naturopathic Physician, I got a preceptorship position at Dr. Gino Tutera's office, now the world-renowned SottoPelle. Being a Naturopathic Physician and believing that the body heals itself, I initially did not like the idea of using hormones to treat menopause. I thought that we were going against the laws of nature. But I stayed, since I was curious to find out what this buzz was all about. I loved helping women feel better. We had women coming to our offices from all over the country and some even from international destinations. I was in my late twenties when I started working there and probably could not relate to all the benefits that women were experiencing from the treatments. Now, ten years later, I swear by this treatment because of the amazing results I've seen.

Bioidentical Hormone Replacement Therapy (BHRT) is different from synthetic hormones. This means that the shape of this hormone is precisely the shape of what your body makes, thus making it bioidentical. It is natural and plant-based. Yams are usually the starting substance. In the lab, they are made into the exact structure of the hormones that our body naturally produces. Our bodies get excited for this missing hormone that is bioidentical and accepts it as its own hormone when this therapy is used. The body responds very well to it rather than to synthetic hormones. They come in different forms, like creams, lozenges, or pellets, which can be implanted under the skin by a trained physician.

As we age, we don't produce enough hormones. Testosterone levels begin to decline in women when they are in their late thirties. It causes symptoms like low energy, anxiety, brain fogginess, low libido, and weight gain.

Then, as we reach closer to menopause, estrogen and progesterone levels decline, which brings on menopause and its classic symptoms of hot flashes, night sweats, mood swings, sleep problems, and vaginal dryness. By choosing to use BHRT, we are not only saving one from not experiencing all these symptoms, but also preventing them from developing chronic diseases like osteoporosis, cardiovascular disease, and breast cancer. One is prone to these diseases when their hormone levels decline as they reach menopause. Does it not make sense to correct the hormone deficiency by natural hormones to prevent these diseases?

At SottoPelle, we specialize in pellet therapy for BHRT. The hormone pellets are implanted under the skin with a minor surgical procedure, and they slowly release the hormones based on the body's need. I learned this method from Dr. Tutera and saw it change people's lives. He was the pioneer who brought the pellet therapy to the US, and I was very fortunate to get the opportunity to learn from and work with the master helping women feel better, optimizing their weight, and helping them have more energy on a day-to-day basis.

Yes, I firmly believe in what I offer my patients and always try the therapies on myself. Since I am in my late thirties now, I use the testosterone alone. I will not need estradiol and progesterone until I get closer to menopause. The testosterone keeps my energy levels high, helps my moods and prevents anxiety, helps to keep my memory sharp and libido good. It also helps to maintain proper muscle mass and burn fat, which most women need!

Premarin is the most commonly prescribed synthetic estrogen. It comes from horses' (mares') urine, which is how it gets its name. Mares (female horse) make 50 different kinds of estrogen, while we make only make three types. With this synthetic hormone, we are introducing foreign substances to our bodies. So if we introduce 50 different estrogens when only three are needed, aren't we increasing our risk to diseases like cancer?

The good news is numerous studies have been done and, in fact, newer studies are constantly published that are in favor of BHRT. Keeping the hormones balanced has many preventative reasons; some of them include maintaining proper bone density and preventing osteoporosis, protection against cardiovascular disease, maintaining good levels of blood sugar, and prevention against breast and colon cancer.

By choosing to use BHRT, we are not only saving women from not experiencing all these symptoms of menopause, but also preventing them from developing chronic diseases like osteoporosis, cardiovascular disease, and breast cancer. If you are prone to these diseases when your hormone levels are declining, then does it not make sense to correct the hormone deficiency by natural hormones to prevent these diseases? Yet you may have heard myths regarding hormone replacement therapy.

Here are five myths about BHRT that need to be busted.

Myth #1: BHRT causes cancer

For healthy adults, BHRT may help reduce the risk of cancer by balancing natural hormone levels. Of course, if someone has a personal history of hormone positive breast cancer, I would not recommend estrogen or progesterone. In fact, testosterone therapy will help them. We have many patients who choose to get testosterone therapy after they have had breast cancer, due to the positive impact it has on their lives.

Myth #2: BHRT causes blood clots

The blood clots myth began when BHRT was first developed, and it stems from the fact that early treatments were not individualized. In fact, the advancements in BHRT allow women to enjoy a healthier post-menopausal stage due to the balance of estrogen, which mitigates the risk of developing coronary artery disease. When a doctor gets a detailed patient history, he/she can determine if a patient has a chance of developing a blood clot. A thrombosis panel can be run to find out any genetic cause for developing clots before recommending BHRT.

Myth #3: BHRT is only recommended during menopause

We have patients in their eighties and a few more in their nineties who get BHRT. These are patients who started the BHRT almost 30 years ago and have decided to continue for the rest of their lives. They not only look 20 years younger than their actual ages, but they act like it too. They have perfect bone density, which their doctors are blown away by. BHRT keeps you from losing your bone density and prevents you from developing osteoporosis, which is common in women after menopause. I like to monitor my patients' bone density via Dexa Scans. I am delighted to share that when a patient has been on our therapy, I almost always notice that their bone density improves every two years when the scan is performed.

Myth #4: BHRT treatments cause hair loss

When estrogen levels decline in a woman, she begins to lose her hair. That is the reason that women start noticing hair loss when they get closer to menopause. By correcting the deficiency using BHRT, we can prevent hair loss. Hair loss is a significant stressor in a woman's lives. No woman that I know of would like to go through it. On the other hand, too much testosterone can cause hair loss. In some women, testosterone converts easily to a form called DHT (Di-hydro Testosterone), which is related to hair loss. Thus, it is the fine hormonal balance that can lead to healthy hair.

Myth #5: BHRT causes weight gain

Testosterone is the hormone that helps us to burn fat and make more muscle. Yes, even women make testosterone naturally and need adequate levels of it to feel good. Of course, we need much fewer amounts compared to men, but don't be of the belief that testosterone is only a male hormone. When testosterone levels drop, we begin to accumulate fat in places where we may not have seen it before. A common place is the mid-abdomen area. Women come to me and say that they have tried every type of diet and exercise but can't seem to lose the weight. They also say that they have never been "so flabby" in their lives. They begin losing muscle tone. By using individualized testosterone therapy, we are able to reverse this.

Honestly, I see that balancing the hormones using BHRT transforms lives. The women tell me that the difference is like night and day. Patients have come back to me with tears of joy and thank me that they got their lives back again. In fact, I have had women's husbands thank me, saying that they got their wives back and a few of them have sent me flowers out of appreciation. All of this says a lot about how the hormones have helped.

Pre-requisites for Treatment

Before I start a patient on this treatment, I review the patient's medical history and have them go for a blood draw to check their hormone levels. We also have the patients do Well Women exams, which include a pap test and breast imaging like a mammogram or ultrasound. I will evaluate every patient on a case by case basis. Based on the patient's lab work, symptoms, medical history, and age, I will determine if the patient is a candidate for this therapy or not. All these tests are another method of ensuring and easing their minds about BHRT.

If someone is the right candidate, BHRT can be offered via different delivery systems. A pharmacy can compound the hormones in the form of a cream, lozenges, or pills. It can also be implanted underneath the skin in the form of pellets. Patients can choose their preferred delivery system.

Then we run a hormone panel before and after the treatments. The lab results and patient's feedback on their symptoms are two things that will help monitor and adjust the treatment. Every patient receives an individualized treatment.

There are some supplements that are valuable in balancing hormone levels and can be used in conjunction with BHRT or by themselves, depending on the need.

1. DIM, or Diindolylmethane, comes from broccoli extract. You can't get this from eating broccoli, as you'd have to eat about a whole bag to get the same amount that you'd get from just one capsule. It's used to help metabolize estrogen better.

   There are two kinds of estrogens: the 2 hydroxy (2OH) and 16 hydroxy (16OH). The 2OH is a kind that we want our estrogen to be converted to. Some women get breast tenderness, which means the body is metabolizing the estrogen to the 16OH, the wrong kind. Why I am stressing this is because if I prescribe estrogen to a woman and she starts to have breast tenderness, putting her on DIM will correct that. Her body will convert it to 2OH, and the tenderness will go away.

2. Calcium D-Glucarate works in a similar way. If there is a build-up of estrogen in a woman's body, or if she is estrogen dominant, Calcium D-Glucarate will help the body eliminate excess estrogen.

People assume symptoms like hair loss, not sleeping at night and exhaustion, and even depression are a part of aging. We assume this is something that we just have to accept, as we did with my grandmother. Yet I have patients who are in their eighties and have been on this therapy for more than 25 years and seen a dramatic difference mentally, physically, and emotionally in their lives. They say that their primary care doctors are blown away by their bone density results. In their eighties, they feel physically strong. Their cognition does not decline, their memory remains sharp, and they have an overall feeling of well-being and good energy levels.

Coming to the US and working with Dr. Tutera and seeing all these benefits from this treatment, I decided that I don't want to go through what my grandmother did. Nor do I want you to go through that as you age. We can take action now and balance your hormones. You can live a happy, healthy, and fulfilled life in every way and at any age.

Adrenal Hormones

Another vital part of your body that affects energy and well-being through these stages are the adrenal glands, which sit on top of the kidneys. The adrenal cortex produces three hormones:

1. Mineralocorticoids: the most important of which is aldosterone. This hormone helps to maintain the body's salt and water levels, which, in turn, regulates blood pressure.

2. Glucocorticoids: predominantly cortisol. This hormone is involved in the response to illness and also helps to regulate body metabolism. Cortisol stimulates glucose production, helping the body to free up the necessary ingredients from storage (fat and muscle) to make glucose. Cortisol also has significant anti-inflammatory effects. In this section, we are mainly going to focus on cortisol and its response to stress.

3. Adrenal androgens: sex hormones mainly DHEA and Testosterone.

The adrenal medulla produces catecholamines. Catecholamines include adrenaline, noradrenaline, and small amounts of dopamine – these hormones are responsible for all the characteristics of the stress response, the so-called 'fight or flight' response.

Handling stress is like handling a bank account – your adrenal bank account. If you have a lot of adrenal reserves, it means that you can spend on the account. Therefore, many people can spend early in life. However, as we grow older, we have to pay more attention to our reserve and replenishment so as to increase those adrenal reserves; we need to live within our means. That means choosing diet, lifestyle, and sleep habits that replenish the reserve.

If you've recently started a new job, started a new school, or moved to a new country, you may feel an enormous amount of pressure and stress, just like I did. Stress affects not only your thyroid, but your adrenal glands, as well as causing you to "burn out." These prolonged periods of stress cause your adrenals to be dysregulated. "The body is no longer able to regulate cortisol levels effectively, which leads to symptoms like fatigue, a lack of enthusiasm, insomnia, and a general lack of vitality" (Hansen, 2017, para. 8). You become exhausted and may start to fall asleep throughout the day, even in public places or while driving your car.

Cortisol levels are generally high in the morning as we wake from a prolonged period of sleep, with an increase of up to fifty percent in the twenty to thirty minutes after waking. This is known as the 'cortisol awakening response'. Then, as the day progresses, our cortisol levels naturally begin to drop in a fairly constant and regular fashion that is termed a diurnal rhythm, ending up as low in the late evening. This allows the body to keep a regular sleeping pattern, with the cortisol level dropping for periods of sleep, then replenishing during the following morning.

The body can also detect and change the timing and cycle of cortisol production and release for certain individuals. A great example is those individuals who work night shifts. In these cases, the pattern and timing of the release of cortisol is reversed to allow for higher levels throughout the late evening and early morning hours. For those of you who travel long distances, a similar rearrangement occurs when we experience jetlag.

Cortisol levels are not just dependent on the time of day. Stress also plays an important role. The exact response depends on the type of stress, whether its short-term acute stress or long-term chronic stress. For short-term stressors like an argument or a fall, we will see a brief spike in cortisol. For longer-term stressors like work stress or illness, we see a consistently higher level of cortisol at all times of the day.

How does all this relate to Adrenal Fatigue? Well, those long-term stressors can eventually deplete the nutrients and precursors that we need to produce cortisol and other hormones. In other words, chronic stress will raise your cortisol levels for a while but, eventually, your body is unable to continue producing cortisol in such high amounts. At this point, we start to see declines in not only cortisol but also key hormones and neurotransmitters like aldosterone, testosterone, epinephrine and more. Additionally, the diurnal rhythm of cortisol production is often disrupted, resulting in late-evening spikes that cause insomnia. (Hansen, 2017)

I recently saw a woman in my practice who basically stayed up the whole night. In the morning, she'd wait to take her daughter to school at around 9 am, and then she'd go to sleep for the day. Her morning cortisol levels were really low and then higher in the evening, giving her a high energy burst at night. This is when one needs help in regulating the diurnal rhythm and balancing cortisol levels with help of botanical medicine and supplements.

We can check for a person's cortisol response by using a salivary test called the Adrenal Stress Index. Refer to the two graphs. The first one shows a normal cortisol response where levels are highest in the morning and gradually declining towards evening. The second graph shows the cortisol response to chronic stress, where cortisol levels have fallen in the morning and are beginning to rise in the night time.

Circadian Cortisol Profile

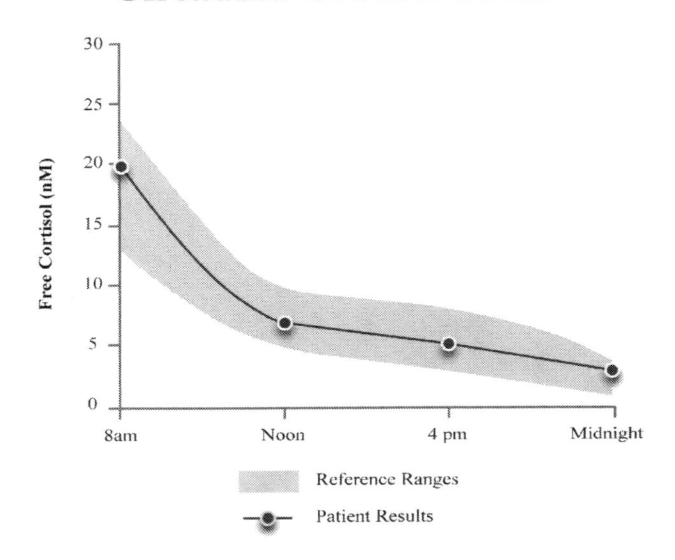

Circadian Cortisol Profile

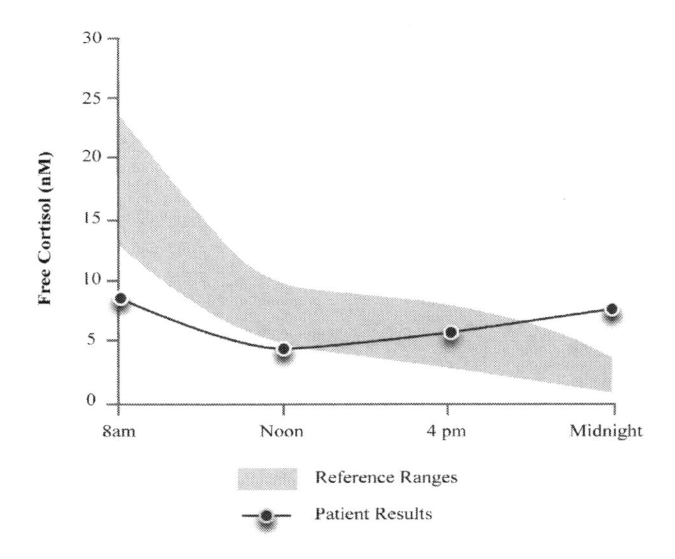

"How can we reverse the effects of long-term stress and regain our energy levels? A combination of good nutrition, supplementation, and effective stress management techniques can quickly result in some significant changes. In the longer term, eliminating the causes of stress is crucial for a full recovery" (Hansen, 2017, para. 9).

The impact of stress is unique to each patient, and it can manifest through a range of symptoms and laboratory values. Comprehensive analysis is required to identify the stress response stage and support each patient's unique needs.

Although specific recommendations differ based on the stage of stress resistance as shown in the table, below are a few considerations:

1. Obtain regular exercise

2. Establish regular bedtimes and obtain sufficient sleep

3. Practice relaxation activities (yoga and meditation)

4. Consider smoking cessation programs

5. Avoid or limit alcohol and sugar consumption

6. Identify and remove food intolerances

	Early Stage	Mid Stage	Late Stage
Symptoms	High stress Anxious or agitated Sleeplessness Tired but wired Higher pulse	Moderate stress Tired	Fatigued/ exhausted Very tired in the evening Difficulty falling asleep and staying asleep Low pulse
Lab Values	Increase in levels of Cortisol, DHEA, Blood Pressure and Blood glucose	Serotonin declines	Decrease in Cortisol, DHEA, Serotonin and Blood pressure
Botanical medicine and supplements	Ashwagandha L-Theanine Magnolia Phosphatidylserine	Rhodiola Holy Basil Eleuthero Ashwagandha Maca	Vit B1 Vit B2 Vit B5 Vit B6 Forskolin Licorice Root **Late stage sleep support** Melatonin Glycine L-Theanine 5- HTP

WHERE TO START?

As you go about your week, try to buy certified organic groceries on your next shopping list and start to create a normal, earlier bedtime routine to help regulate your adrenals.

If you think you are starting menopause or have any of the symptoms mentioned above, talk to your doctor about balancing your hormones. You can ask him or her for a complete hormone evaluation, like explained in this chapter. These simple steps will increase your day-to-day energy and help you avoid burnout, plus elevate your mood.

STEP 6: EMOTIONAL HEALING

In 2016, I had the worst experience of my life.

Today, I am thankful for that experience, since it helped me reset my priorities. It made me stop and rethink my life. I understood how I had allowed people to take advantage of me in big and small ways before. I have a very giving and caring heart, which makes me put people before myself. But with this experience, I was so badly hurt that I could not continue living the way I was, and it helped me put a lot of things into perspective. That traumatic experience changed my life, but how I responded to it helped me heal emotionally. I can really say I finally grew up at the age of 38!

I did not realize that I was wasting a lot of my precious time and energy pleasing others while hurting my own self. Yet today, I am thankful to all these people in the past that took advantage of me, since it's because of them that I have learned my life lessons. I'm stronger now. With this strength, I have found time to write this book and not feed energy vampires! Yes, that is what they are called. I learned about this term when I heard a talk by Dr. Christiane Northrup.

Stress is your body's way of protecting itself from danger, real or imagined. Short-term stress can be helpful, like giving you an increase of hormones, such as adrenaline and cortisol, that will help you finish your school paper or help you feel the need to pay your bills on time. However, long-term stress, like the experience I had in 2016, has been linked to health conditions.

Your thyroid and adrenals affect your mood. Stress increases damage to the thyroid and increases symptoms of leaky gut, which then causes inflammation in your brain. You then have mood changes, like aggression or sadness. There are plenty of times in conventional medicine when a patient is put on one medication for a mood disorder and then another if that one doesn't work. The symptoms are suppressed when, really, a patient may have something going on beyond a mood disorder. It goes back to treating the root cause of a problem rather than the symptoms. And all this is aggravated by stress.

Realizing the kind of emotional person you are, what kind of energies others have, and learning to focus and cope with stress is an important step to heal not only your thyroid, but your soul as well.

HOW TO TELL IF YOU'RE AN EMPATH

Knowing your emotional personality will help you discover a better way to treat your mental well-being and transfer this over to your physical health as well. To your thyroid.

Over time, I realized I am an empath, and I do think that there are many people in this world who are similar to me. Therefore, I want to dedicate a section of my book to this personality type.

There is a spectrum of sensitivity that exists in human beings. Empaths are emotional sponges who absorb both the stress and joy of the world. Dr. Judith Orloff says in her book, The Empath's Survival Guide, "We feel everything, often to an extreme, and have little guard up between others and ourselves. As a result, we are often overwhelmed by excessive stimulation and are prone to exhaustion and sensory overload" (p. 1). I came across the word "empath" when I listened to Dr. Christiane Northrup's video. She talked about energy vampires and how they get attracted to us and drain our energy.

There are different types of energy vampires, and they love us, since we are very kind, compassionate, and caring. We feel that everyone else is also like us and feels the same emotions, but that is not true. Narcissists are one of the energy vampires that we need to stay away from, since they are cold-hearted and would like to use us to meet their needs. Narcissists will attract empaths like a moth to a flame.

Traits of an Empath

You may have some traits of being an empath yourself. I will help you identify if you are an empath, discuss some types of energy vampires, provide you with life protection strategies and grounding techniques to help you successfully survive in this world. Before I begin, let me tell you to enjoy this precious gift of being an empath, since you have the ability to sense and live your life with full passion. Ashley Aliff mentions some of these traits and more on her site, The Awakened Mind.

1. Feeling other people's emotions and taking them on as your own. This is a huge one for empaths. To some, they will feel emotions of those nearby, and with others, they will feel emotions from those a vast distance away.
2. They can tell when someone is not honest: If a friend or a loved one is telling you lies, you know it (although many empaths try not to focus on this because knowing a loved one is lying can be painful). Or if someone is saying one thing but feeling/thinking another, you know.
3. Others will want to offload their problems on you, even strangers: An empath can become a dumping ground for everyone else's issues and problems, which, if they're not careful can end up as their own.

4. Constant fatigue: Empaths often get drained of energy, either from energy vampires or just taking on too much from others, which even sleep will not cure.
5. Creative: From singing, dancing, acting, drawing, or writing, an empath will have a strong creative streak and a vivid imagination.
6. Love of nature and animals: Being outdoors in nature is a must for empaths and pets are an essential part of their life.
7. Need for solitude: An empath will go stir-crazy if they don't get quiet time. This is even obvious in empathic children.
8. Gets bored or distracted easily if not stimulated: Work, school, and home life has to be kept interesting for an empath, or they switch off from it and end up daydreaming.
9. Strives for the truth: This becomes more prevalent when an empath discovers his/her gifts and birthright. Anything untruthful feels plain wrong.
10. Likes adventure, freedom and travel: Empaths are free spirits.
11. Prone to carry weight without necessarily overeating: The excess weight is a form of protection to stop the negative incoming energies from having as much impact.
12. They are drawn to holistic and healing therapies.

13. Knowing: Empaths know stuff without being told. It's a knowing that goes way beyond intuition or gut feelings.
14. Being in public places can be overwhelming: Places like shopping malls, supermarkets, or stadiums where there are lots of people around can fill the empath with turbulently vexed emotions that are coming from others.

If you can say yes to most or all of the above, then you are most definitely an empath.

Some relations are positive and energizing for empaths, but others are draining. In fact, some people can suck the positivity and peacefulness right out of you. The super toxic ones can make you believe that you are flawed and unlovable. Fear and insecurity motivate these drainers. They annoy and deplete many people, not just you.

Of all the vampires, narcissists can be the most destructive to empaths. They act as if the world revolves around them. They need to be the center of attention and require endless praise. They can do much damage to empaths because they have little or no capacity for unconditional love. If you don't do things their way or if you disagree with them, they become cold and punishing, withhold love, or give you the silent treatment, which can last days or weeks.

Empaths are compassionate and expect others to be the same, so they make the mistake of trying to win over a narcissist with love. That is not going to work. It's like expecting someone without a heart to know how to love.

And with these unhealthy situations, an empath can become overly stressed. But here are a few techniques to help you protect yourself from energy vampires and stress, thus improving your overall health.

Cord-cutting visualization is a technique you can use to protect yourself from narcissists, a way to help ease the pain of ending the relationship. "In a calm state, picture cords of light connecting both of you. Inwardly say thank you for what you've learned from the relationship, even if the lessons were hard. Then firmly assert, "It's time to break our bonds completely." Next, visualize taking a pair of scissors and cutting each bond so that you are free of any energetic ties" (Orloff, 2017, para. 3). This may feel strange, but physical gestures help.

Shielding visualization is a quick way to protect yourself that many empaths rely on, to block out toxic energy while allowing the flow of positive energy.

The minute you're uncomfortable with a person, a place, or a situation, put up your shield. Allow five minutes for this exercise. Begin by taking a few deep, long breaths. Breathe in, and then exhale, letting out a big exhalation. Feel the sensuality of the breath, the connection to prana, or sacred life force. Now visualize a shield of white or pink light that surrounds your body completely. This shield protects you from anything negative, stressful, toxic or unwelcome. Within the protection of this shield, feel centered, happy and energized. Internally say, "Thank you for this protection."

Empaths have much to offer. Don't let your sensitivities wear you down. Instead, embrace the gifts of being an empath and learn strategies to ground yourself. We must all do our part to contribute to this beautiful world and make it a better place for everyone.

HOW TO DEAL WITH STRESS OR EMOTIONAL TRAUMA

I'd like to move on to how to deal with stress or emotional trauma for everyone, empath or not.

When families get together, there can either be excitement and happiness or there can be anger, fear, and resentment, which I am sure you have felt at your last Thanksgiving or Christmas party. Our emotional reactions depend upon our past experiences in our relationships. As human beings, we sometimes torment ourselves about choices we've made, words we've spoken, and the path not taken. These thoughts and judgments are the sources of our emotional pain.

"While the body spontaneously lets go of pain the moment the underlying cause is healed, the mind has a mysterious instinct for holding on. Through the mind, we create a prison of suffering and then forget that we are the architect and that we ourselves hold the key that will set us free."

– Deepak Chopra

Even after years of emotional healing work, we all sometimes make the mistake of believing that something out there makes us angry, depressed, anxious, or afraid. In reality, outside events are only triggers. The cause of every emotion is within ourselves. We cause our own stress.

By uncovering the false perceptions that cause us to cling to pain, we can open to a deep experience of peace. Yes, there are all kinds of people out there. Some of them are toxic and manipulate other people according to their whims and wishes and cause emotional trauma and abuse. It is hard to recognize emotional abuse compared to physical abuse, since there are no scars or bruises seen physically. The victim in this case firstly needs to realize the situation they are in before they can seek help. In most cases of emotional abuse, the victim may be in denial since they may have lived with this abuse for a very long time.

I would like to share some natural ways to help people with emotional trauma and relieve stress.

Homeopathy works beautifully in this case. It is a practice of medicine that also involves the artistic skill of the physician to find the best remedy for the patient. The impact that homeopathy has on the emotional plane of a person can be life-changing. I have used it successfully to treat patients with mental-emotional issues like anxiety and depression.

Essential oils are very effective. The aroma can lift moods significantly. They are either available as single oils or in blends; it depends on the purpose for which you are using it. They can be directly applied to the skin or added to a diffuser to spread the aroma in the room. I recommend using lavender, rose, and frankincense for anxiety. I have been using the one called "Live with Passion" by Young Living. I have a deep passion for the medicine I practice and like to help as many people as possible in different ways. So using this oil enhances this feeling in me.

Journaling and penning down your thoughts is a great therapeutic tool. You can either choose to do it every night while sipping hot chamomile tea or do it from time to time. I do it as needed. There have been certain times in my life that have been more challenging, and I needed to write more regularly. I have journaled for years, and it helps me go back years and self-reflect. I can identify patterns of how my reactions were to certain situations and helps me learn how to change what I don't like. It also helps me realize what matters to me and helps me reinstate my morals and values.

Meditation helps you find your true self and purpose in life. It brings mental peace and increases awareness. There are many different kinds of meditations available. If you have never tried it before, you must start with a short seven- to ten-minute guided meditation.

YouTube can be your friend as well. I encourage you to try the 21 days meditation by Oprah and Deepak Chopra. You can register by email and can download the app on your phone. It is free. Their recent meditation is about creating peace from inside out. They talk about the three ancient Indian practices that help immensely:

Seva

Focuses on the spiritual connection that is developed with the world when we offer selfless service to others. Not only do we help others through our service, but we also gain spiritually in joy and compassion, and that lifts us up as well. Some examples are doing weekly volunteer work at a hospital or feeding the homeless people.

Sadhana

It translates to "a means to accomplish something." The word "your" is significant here because everyone's journey into self-awakening is unique. You each have your own spiritual path and Sadhana is a practice or routine that will help you find your way. Along the way, you must learn how to trust in yourself - in your inner strength, courage, and inspiration.

Satsang

When you connect with others who also hold a vision of world peace, compassion, and human dignity, you are magnifying the power of your positive influence in the world many times over. This is the power of spiritual community or Satsang. It could be attending church or a temple on Sundays or be part of a community group like Chinmaya Mission where you go as a family to learn, grow, and share with like-minded people.

Dr. Low Dog's 4-7-8 Breath Meditation Exercise

Take a moment and breathe!

Researchers have shown that by altering the rhythm of our breath, we can have a powerful effect on our emotions. It's one of the best tools we have to counteract the effects of stress. The easiest way to do it is to sit comfortably in a chair, feet on the floor, hands on your knees, and inhale for the count of four, hold your breath for the count of seven, and then exhale for the count of eight. If you do this four times, every morning, and every night, or when you feel like you're in a stressful situation, I promise you, it will help calm you, center you.

After you finish the series, you'll feel much better prepared to enter back into your world. Breathwork is a powerful tool, it doesn't cost you anything, and you can take it with you wherever you go.

HOW TO FOCUS AND RE-ENERGIZE

There are days when we are physically tired or days when our emotions or feelings take over. Women, you all especially know what I am talking about, don't you? What can we do to stay motivated and move in the direction of our goals?

I say mind over matter.

Thus, let our minds remind us over and over so that we can stay focused, centered, and get that task accomplished, whatever it may be. Even though I believe in mind over matter, it is hard to stay in the zone at all times because many things happen around you all day. Like things that happen at your workplace, or your child's school, or what you hear on the news, etc. I would like to share with you a few things and practices that can help you stay inspired, centered and focused on your path.

Inspiration Corner: Create a space in your home that inspires you. You can dedicate a space or a corner in your bedroom to it. Add things to that area which are meaningful for you.

For example, I have a bookshelf in my room that is made from unprocessed wood of pine trees grown in Show Low, Arizona. It is meaningful to me since it's made from wood in its natural form and it is handmade by someone that I personally know. She provides custom orders. Please check out her website at **http://mountaingirlscreations.com/**

Besides my favorite collection of books, my bookshelf holds things that are inspiring to me and are gifted by special people in my life. There is a sign that says "DREAM." It reminds me to live my dream every day, which I do through my work. A crystal tree that upon shaking brings Sedona's powerful vortex energy to me. It reminds me to be surrounded by good and positive energy.

A special friend gifted me crystal bracelets that were charged by her aunt using moonlight. Each one of them has a different purpose. I feel that I stay more grounded when I wear them. I have pictures of my husband and boys, so when I see them, my heart instantly fills up with love. The Symbol of Om, which is the universal sound and is the essential vibration of creation reminds me to stay centered and at peace. In this way, my inspiration corner adds meaning to my life and provides constant reminders to follow my passion and stay on my path.

"Joy" is one of the essential oils by Young Living. It works best when you rub a few drops over your heart. My medical assistant and I use it when we are having a hard day at work. The patients for the rest of the day smell the aroma, and we all stay in a joyful mood. You may think that it is a placebo effect. I would say give it a try for yourself and see.

Golden Hour: Dr. Shivangi Maletia Jangra says that we should wake up at 5 am and dedicate an hour to be by ourselves. Rather than grabbing our phone first thing in the morning to check Facebook or Whatsapp, do the following:

In that Golden Hour, recharge your Mind, Body, and Soul, dedicating 20 minutes to each.

For your Mind — Meditate for 20 minutes. Focus on your breathing. Find the stillness. Let any thoughts that come to your mind pass by gently. You can play meditation music or do guided meditations.

For your Body — Exercise for 20 minutes. I recommend yoga poses; develop a flow and practice Surya Namaskars. You can vary your exercise routine during days of the week. You can incorporate some cardio exercises by using DVDs or YouTube. There are dance workouts available if that is what you enjoy. There are so many options to choose from that there should never be an excuse.

For your Soul — Read something that inspires you for 20 minutes. I enjoy books by Brendon Burchard, and I am currently reading his book called High Performance Habits. I also like books by Robin Sharma, Don Miguel Ruiz, and Swami Chinmayananda.

Imagine how ready you will be to start your day if you practice Golden Hour every morning. You will be prepared to take on any challenge that comes your way and deal with it peacefully with a steady mind.

Mason Jar Gratitude Notes: Buy a mason jar and keep it in your family room. When anyone in the family has something pleasant happen to them, have them write a note about it and drop it in the jar. During the year, see the jar fill up. At the end of the year, over the holiday time, sit with your family and read all the notes. There will be so much to be thankful for.

Take small and simple steps to make a good life. Remember, the trinity of life comprises body, mind, and soul. You need to be balanced at all three levels to achieve and enjoy optimal health. I truly believe that if we have a heart full of love, compassion, and kindness, then that is what we will attract. It will bring inner peace. Love is the only reason for our existence.

Since learning how stress affects me, how I am an empath, and how to cope with stress, I have implemented these coping methods and have become a less stressed and more focused person. My thyroid levels have improved, and I feel more like myself, though it wasn't always easy. I've had to break some friendships as well, some that had lasted for long years. It broke my heart. This is difficult for anyone to do and was a big deal for me as well.

But I decided I must be happy in my center because I want to be the healer, to give and take care of people like you. If I am not happy, I can't take care of you. The happy and healthy mind leads to a healthy body, including your thyroid. Don't let stress get you down. Let life be simple.

WHERE TO START?

Emotional healing and learning how to cope with stress is not only good for your thyroid, but for peace in your life. For your soul. While I recommend all the methods mentioned in this chapter, to start, I would say try Dr. Low Dog's breathing exercise. Breath is essential for life and for calming yourself down. When your child is angry, have you ever told them just to breathe? You can fight your anger and stress with simple breathing exercises as well. Also, try the Golden Hour and have a moment to yourself. You need time to remember who you are and what's important for you in your life.

STEP 7:

THE WHOLE PICTURE

The last step to a healthy thyroid is to really understand the whole picture, which is crucial, as it is one of the six fundamental principles of Naturopathic Medicine, Treat the Whole Person.

Here's a little recap of the Seven Steps to Heal your Thyroid.

1. Understanding Your Thyroid

Knowing how your thyroid works is a great first step to understanding and healing your thyroid. You wouldn't want to try and fix a car engine without knowing how it works first, right?

2. Naturopathic Treatments

If you find out you have a thyroid problem, the standard treatment is to give you the medicine and send you on your way. Now you know and understand that there are so many more options out there for you not just in treatment, but in prevention as well.

3. Heal Your Gut

Health begins in your gut. Not only are you what you eat, but you are also what you absorb and digest. Knowing the right foods that work for your unique body will not only heal your thyroid, but help you lose weight as well.

4. Reduce Toxic Environmental Exposure

The world we live in has become a toxic place, from the foods we eat to our environment, yet it can be prevented. Shop on the outside aisles of your grocery store and buy organic food whenever possible.

5. Balancing Your Hormones

Hormones are the messengers of our body's own endocrine system. They are natural. When we are deficient in them, we can experience difficult symptoms. We can reverse this by correcting this deficiency by using natural, plant-based bioidentical hormones. I have seen them change lives; they can change yours.

6. Emotional Healing

Stress affects your adrenals and thyroid; it upsets the balance in your body and is a cause of depression. Knowing how to prevent stress and learn coping methods will lead you on your path to a healthy thyroid and a happy and simple life.

7. Treat the Whole Person

In Naturopathic Medicine, we don't treat different parts of the body, but rather, consider the whole person. Their physical makeup, the symptoms they are having, how they are doing emotionally, and spiritually is important to understand. A cardiologist treats people with heart issues or a dermatologist treats people with skin issues. There is definitely a need for medical specialties like Cardiology, Gastroenterology, Dermatology, etc., but sometimes if we treat the body in parts, we can miss out on addressing some key aspects.

Of course, you wouldn't want an electrician to look at your toilet, same as you wouldn't want the plumber to fix your roof. It would be a disaster. Professionals are needed in their area, and we wouldn't do well without them. However, we cannot forget to look at the root cause of your problem or illness and correct it, rather than just the symptoms. You wouldn't want that same plumber to merely place a bandage on a leak and walk away, would you? You'd want the cause of the problem fixed. That's what I do. A Naturopathic Doctor identifies and treats the root cause of the problem.

For example, I had a patient come to me who had suffered from cystic acne for 20 years. She was a beautiful woman, but her acne was affecting her self-esteem, and thus,her everyday life. She had seen every dermatologist that she was referred to but no-one was able to cure her acne. She had tried every commercial product, home remedy, topical and oral medicine for acne. She even tried dietary changes and stress management, yet nothing helped.

After ordering comprehensive labs, I figured out that she had a hormonal imbalance. Her testosterone levels were high. This can happen in the case of Polycystic Ovarian Syndrome, when ovaries make cysts that produce androgens. This increases testosterone levels and can cause acne, unwanted body hair, hair loss, and irregular cycles. I balanced her high testosterone by prescribing bioidentical natural estradiol cream and her 20-year-long acne problem resolved. She was ecstatic. She said that she no longer woke up to find 20 blemishes to cover and she could finally roam around make-up free.

At last, she received the results she dreamed of and felt like herself again. With Naturopathic Medicine, we are treating the problem rather than just muting or fighting the symptoms. I don't want you to just feel better, but heal you from the inside out.

This is why it's so important to look at the whole picture.

TRINITY OF LIFE: MIND, BODY & SOUL

One way to treat you as a whole person and not just treat the labs or symptoms is to understand and use the concept of Trinity of Life. To reach true happiness, we must have harmony and balance, not only with our hormones, but our body, mind, and soul.

1. Mind

"Watch your thoughts, for they become words.
Watch your words, for they become actions.
Watch your actions, for they become...habits.
Watch your habits, for they become your character.
And watch your character, for it becomes your destiny!
What we think we become."

-Margaret Thatcher

Life is about the choices we make—not just the large decisions like which career to make or who to marry, but the little everyday choices. It starts in the morning, with what time you choose to wake up. Will you hit the snooze button? Will you get up early and start with a meditation? Whichever you choose is the foundation for the rest of your day, and thus, your week, month, and life. As the common saying goes, will your glass be half empty or half full? A positive attitude or a mind filled with good thoughts can change the course of your life simply with how you handle stress and relationships.

A positive mind can improve your health.

One way to keep a positive attitude is to surround yourself with like-minded people. It is best to avoid and even cut off relationships with people who are energy vampires or narcissists, hard as it may be. In the end, you must think about what is right for you and those you love. My motivation was to be able to help people like you, which I couldn't do if bad relationships were weighing me down and sucking away my energy. Find people who you connect with, people with whom you share not only hobbies, but humor as well. Create positive energy together.

If you break off a relationship as I did in 2016, you may find yourself dwelling on the past. Bad thoughts can enter your mind, maybe even doubting yourself if it was the right decision. Humans tend to remember the bad and focus on it instead of thinking of the good. Thoughts are always coming to the mind; let the negative ones pass by. Don't dwell on the past or bad thoughts, otherwise they will build up into this giant ball and weigh you down.

2. Body

Perhaps you've been pregnant. Do you remember what it felt like? There were many nights you couldn't sleep because you couldn't get your leg or belly into the right position and then when you did, you needed to use the restroom.

Walking was difficult, as was tying your shoelaces. Pregnancy, while obviously natural, is a time of difficult symptoms that interfere with your quality of life. How much would you have paid at one point to have a decent night's sleep? Or to rid yourself of the labor pain? You can have all the wealth in the world, but without health, you can't enjoy life.

To ensure your body's health long into old age, you must consistently exercise, take the right kind of supplements that absorb well into the body, and eat the right type of food. Exercise without overdoing it. You can find an excellent resource of workouts on YouTube if you don't have the time to go to a gym or class. Take supplements, such as your multivitamin, that will increase your body's overall health. Find out your food sensitivities to avoid leaky gut and inflammation and reduce toxic environmental exposure. Basically, use this book as a stepping stone to better health.

Treat your body with respect now so it will respect you later.

3. Soul

Without the soul, our bodies cannot live. Our soul is the driving force behind every movement, breath & action. You must take care of your soul to find a balance and joy in your life. There are a few ways to do this.

I believe in Oneness. God is present in many

different forms, but there is One Superpower. How you chose to love, praise, or think about that Superpower is up to you.

You can begin your Golden Hour routine with some inspirational reading. This could be a good book that you enjoy, a magazine that inspires you, or a spiritual book that you believe in. This will help your day get started focusing on some positive thoughts, plus helps you sleep better at night. Your inspirational reading will create a calm and peaceful soul.

You can create an inspiration corner that has meaning to you. A place of your own that captures a bit of your essence and personality. You can put your inspirational quotes and books, pictures or souvenirs from loved ones, and spiritual symbols. This will help induce a happy mind and provide reminders to follow your passion. Knowing who you are can help your soul find peace. You can also make this corner or area a place where you practice humility and bow to your altar in prayer. You can try the Golden Hour by Dr. Shivangi MaletiaJangra. Wake up at 5 am and have some time alone to yourself. Bow down to your altar and be thankful for another beautiful day. Light an incense stick that fills up the room with natural aromas.

A FINAL WHERE TO START

A Recap to Increase Energy, Elevate Mood, & Optimize Weight

Since my desire is to make sure you are able to understand each of these steps to having a healthy thyroid and balanced life, I'd like to give you one final "Where to Start," a summary of sorts to remind you exactly how you can increase your energy, elevate your mood, and optimize your weight. To look at the book as a whole, kind of like we'd do for a patient.

If you are suffering and having to push yourself every day, I want to let you know that you don't need to live like that anymore. I want you to take action. Thus, I am going to recap what you can do and, importantly, which functional tests to order to give you the best information to find the root cause of the problem.

Increase Your Energy

Coffee, energy drinks, and foods that claim to increase your energy are everywhere for a reason. We have become a society, especially in the United States, of people who must hustle and always be productive to the point of burnout. We crave more energy to simply get through the day.

Women, you know all about stress. You have the physical energy of lifting kids into car seats, go to work, the stress pregnancy and monthly hormonal changes add to your body. Then there's the mental energy in taking care of your family, work, and your to-do list. These two forms, mental and physical energy, need to be refilled daily, and this can be done using the steps mentioned in this book.

Remember, your health relates back to your gut. Food is energy, so making sure you make healthy food choices is vital. The food choices you make and how often you eat will directly impact your energy. Eat balanced meals that provide all the three macronutrients, good carbs from multi-colored veggies and fruits, healthy fats like avocados, nuts and coconut oil, and a lean protein. Eating five to six small meals a day keeps one's metabolism and energy levels up, unlike choosing an energy drink to kill your appetite, which not only gives you short bursts of energy but will eventually lead to adrenal fatigue if you start depending on them.

With your macronutrient-balanced diet, always consider the micronutrients. Micronutrients, such as vitamins, minerals, and antioxidants, work at the cellular level and are directly related to the production of energy by running our biochemical pathways. So consider doing the Micronutrient Test that I mentioned in Step 2 to find out what your cells need and thus personalize your treatment.

Your energy depends on how good your sleep is at night. Do you wake up rested or do you need a cup of coffee to get you going? Are you dragging during the day and wired-up at night? If you have any of these symptoms, definitely consider doing a hormone panel. I have explained the Complete Thyroid Panel in Step 1 and Adrenal Panel in Step 5. The saliva-based comprehensive adrenal test is called Adrenal Stress Index.

We also talked about heavy metal testing. Knowing the toxins or metals in you may help to decide if they are causing a depletion of your energy levels by unbalancing your hormones, thus affecting your thyroid.

Regular exercising keeps your energy levels up. There is no excuse for not having time to exercise. There are so many options to choose from, like jogging at your neighborhood park, taking a yoga class, joining a gym, and if you cannot find even twice a week to commit to this, then follow some YouTube videos in the comfort of your home.

Women and men nearing their forties begin to complain of low energy. At this point in life, make sure that you check your testosterone hormone levels. Yes, it is as important in women as it is in men. Testosterone deficiency is directly related to the drop in your energy.

Mental energy is vital to your overall health as well. Since stress affects your thyroid and adrenals, it is important to learn how to cope with your stress in order to preserve your energy. A little reminder: A good place to start to relieve the worries in your mind is by practicing meditation, mason jar gratitude notes, journaling, and walking or jogging out in nature.

You can be an energetic person well into old age. I have many patients who are in their eighties and have the energy of someone much younger. It's possible for you too.

Elevate Your Mood

You want to live a life full of energy with a body that you feel comfortable in, but your mood is what controls your overall happiness. While the seven steps we've covered will help you to have a better mood, happiness first comes from within. Life and circumstances certainly get in the way, but when you wake up in the morning, you have a choice to either work to your best ability to be happy or to let the world take control of you and your desires. Mind over matter. Here's a reminder of areas of this book that will help you make that morning choice to be happy.

While meditation is part of you gaining your mental energy, it also goes with calming your mind and increases awareness. It helps you find your true purpose in life. Indecision causes much of life's stress; meditation enables you to find those answers in your life. You can try a few forms that I use: the 21 Day Meditation series with Oprah and Deepak Chopra, and Dr. Low Dog's 4-7-8 Breath Meditation Exercise.

Exercise, while necessary for optimizing your weight, also increases your energy and elevates your mood. Each time you exercise, you increase your serotonin, which is a neurotransmitter that creates that happy feeling. Drugs like heroin and meth increase serotonin levels to get that high and joyful feeling, but you can also accomplish this through healthy means like being in nature and exercise. It can be hard to start but going for a walk at a nearby park or going to the gym will help you feel like yourself again. Your daily or weekly workout may become your hobby, but it is a good idea to have another hobby that interests you as well, like dancing was for me as a child.

Kids love sweets. Their smile as you hand them a colorful, sugary treat alone can increase your serotonin and boost your spirits, yet sugar is a cause of mood fluctuations. The sugar rush may help you feel in a good mood momentarily, but remember, the crash that follows right after will leave you craving for more. The vicious cycle continues, and you begin to get dependent on something that is causing inflammation in your body besides adding the pounds. Eating a balanced diet, including five to six small meals helps to keep your blood sugar under control and your moods stable.

Another way to elevate your mood, especially as you go through certain stages in your life, post 35 years of age, is to consider BHRT. It is the time when hormones begin to fluctuate and along with that bring along symptoms that affect your mood, like depression and anxiety. Consider this natural form of hormone replacement therapy to help you stabilize your moods so that everyone in your family and people you work with stay happy as well!

Your thyroid has a direct connection with the brain and the area that controls your mood, thus optimizing the thyroid is one of the most important ways to elevate your mood. Remember, our thyroid gland is our master gland for metabolism. So if the thyroid is slow, then everything in our body is slow, including the low moods, causing depression. Adrenal health plays as critical role in how you feel. People with adrenal fatigue feel depressed and sluggish. Thus, we need correct testing and then appropriate treatments to help the mood and overall health.

Optimize Your Weight

These days, our world is filled with diet and fads that will help you lose ten pounds in two weeks or something along those lines. Diets seem exciting, especially when you want to lose weight quickly for a special occasion. Yet, as you've learned, there is no perfect diet. Each person's body is different and should be treated as such.

While Paleo diet or the Keto diet may seem like healthy diet choices, your body may not agree with it. You may have a food sensitivity to one of the foods suggested like my patient did with eggs when she was following the Paleo diet and ended up gaining weight. Yet there are ways to help you become healthy and naturally lose weight as we address the root cause of your problem.

Remember, your health depends on your gut, including your weight. I highly recommend you do the GI Map Test to find out the status of your microbiome. We have trillions of microorganisms in our gut, and we want to make sure that they are living in harmony. Overgrowth of any micro organisms is going to give rise to a host of symptoms which will affect our digestion and thus our weight. Stay away from common food allergies or better yet, find a Naturopathic Doctor like me who can order functional medicine testing like GI Map, Food Sensitivity, and a Genetic Weight Management Panel. Once we have this vital information, then we can personalize your treatment.

Make healthy choices in food, in general. Eat organic and GMO-free. Avoid toxin exposures from the environment as much as possible. Follow the Clean 15 and avoid the Dirty Dozen lists that you will find at ***www.ewg.org***. Eat plant-based foods like broccoli or brusselsprouts that will support your living to help remove unavoidable toxins you've built up in your body from your environment. Eat food in its natural forms and avoid the processed foods that come in boxes and cans. Remember, if your great-grandfather didn't eat it, neither should you.

Exercise is an integral part of any plan to lose weight. You can find great YouTube videos or DVDs that provide excellent exercise routines if finding time to exercise is a challenge, or you are a busy mom who is multi-tasking. Yoga is also a wonderful form of exercise that will give you an overall workout while calming your mind and energizing your spirit. You can join a local gym and take different classes, like Zumba, Tabata, or hip-hop. Work with a personal trainer or coach who can work with your individual needs. Go out for a walk or jog and breathe some fresh air and connect with nature. Move that body, stay lean, and feel good.

One of the symptoms of Hashimoto's and hypothyroidism is weight gain because your metabolism slows down. I noticed a significant change in my weight when I was first diagnosed. I couldn't fit into my clothes, and even my friends could see the difference. Yet, once I optimized my thyroid by following the seven steps, my weight dropped, and I felt like myself again.

This is also true with your adrenals. Like we discussed, adrenal fatigue is caused by stress and lack of healthy lifestyle choices, including lack of sleep and wrong foods. This causes burnout and can make you feel depressed and sluggish, which in turn causes you to make worse food choices and not exercise. Balancing your adrenals and optimizing your thyroid will optimize your weight.

A FINAL CALL TO ACTION

As a child, you may have dreamed of being an astronaut, ballerina, or even a saint. I dreamt of serving others, just like my grandfather. To change the world by serving you. While we should follow our inspirations and paths, sometimes as we grow up, we just wish to live a healthy and simple life. And life can be simple. The steps we have covered will help you to not only have a healthy thyroid but help you walk around in a body and weight you feel comfortable in, to have enough energy and elevate your mood. A balance of mind, body, and soul.

But here is the catch. This entire book comes down to one simple fact: **It is Your Choice**.

You can keep eating processed or dirty foods that hurt your gut. There doesn't need to be a corner in your home for your emotional healing, and you may think it isn't necessary to be tested for food sensitivities or replace your hormones. And you'd be right. You don't need to do any of this. But the thyroid affects every part of your body; thus, if you ignore it, you will not be balanced and therefore unhappy. Happiness is a choice. Health is a choice.

What do you choose?

Yet, while the choice to be healthy and happy is yours, you don't have to go through your path alone. I have made it my destiny to help women like you. Like Mother Teresa, I want to help people one by one, to cause a small ripple in the pond of humanity.

You can reach out to a Naturopathic or Functional Medicine Doctor who will not only treat your symptoms but treat you as a whole person. I have been in your place. I know what it's like to struggle and push yourself every day without knowing what's wrong with your body. I know what it's like to deny there is something wrong because you just don't want to admit it. But if you choose to be healthy, if you realize you may have a problem and you decide you want someone to guide you, I can be your teacher. A mentor that goes on even past these pages.

I have met amazing people in my life path, famous and not, yet you never know when a saint will walk through your door, or someone who will change your life.

Will you walk through my door?

REFERENCES

STEP 1:
UNDERSTANDING YOUR THYROID

Bunevicius, R. et al. (1999). Effects of thyroxine as compared with thyroxine plus triiodothyronine in patients with hypothyroidism.New England Journal of Medicine. 340(6), 424-9.

STEP 2:
NATUROPATHIC TREATMENTS

Barman, D.(2014-2016). Micronutrient testing. Retrieved from:

http://www.thymeforyounutrition.com/mnt-overview.html

Gorres G et al. Bone mineral density in patients receiving suppressive doses of thyroxine for differentiated thyroid carcinoma Eur J Nucl Med 1996 Ann. Int. Med. 2000; 132:270-278.

Hak, EA, Pols H, Visser TJ, et al. Subclinical hypothyroidism is an independent risk factor for atherosclerosis and myocardial infarction in elderly women: The Rotterdam Study.

Hamilton MA, Stevenson LW, Fonarow, G.C., et al. Safety and Hemodynamic Effects of Intravenous Triiodothyronine in Advanced Congestive Heart Failure. American Journal of Cardiology. 1998 Feb 15; 81(4)443-447.

Hoang, T.D., et al. (2013). Desiccated thyroid extract compared with levothyroxine in treatment of hypothyroidism: a randomized, double-blind, crossover study. The Journal of Clinical Endocrinology & Metabolism. 98(5), 1982-90.

Kelly, T. A favourable risk-benefit analysis of high dose thyroid for treatment of bipolar disorders with regard to osteoporosis. J Affect Disord. 2014 Sep; 166:353-8.

Natural On (n.d.).14 best herbs for thyroid problems and support for healthy thyroids. Retrieved from:

https://naturalon.com/14-best-herbs-for-thyroid-problems-and-support-for-healthy-thyroids/view-all/

Osansky, E. (2012). 3 herbs which can help with hyperthyroidism. Natural Endocrine Solutions. Retrieved from:

http://www.naturalendocrinesolutions.com/articles/3-herbs-which-can-help-with-hyperthyroidism/

Pure Encapsulations (2016). Retrieved from:

https://www.pureencapsulations.com/media/Nrf2%20Detox.pdf

Razvi S et al. The influence of age on the relationship between subclinical hypothyroidism and ischemic heart disease: a meta-analysis. J Clin Endocrinol Metab. 2008 Aug; 93(8): 2998-3007 6

Thyroid Advisor (n.d.). Effects of kelp for thyroid. Retrieved from:

https://thyroidadvisor.com/effects-kelp-thyroid/

STEP 3: HEAL YOUR GUT

Diagnostic Solutions Laboratory (2017). The GI Microbial Assay Plus (GI-MAP). Quantitative PCR Stool Technology for the Integrative and Functional Medicine Practitioner. Retrieved from:

https://www.diagnosticsolutionslab.com/sites/default/files/gi-map-white-paper-01-2018.pdf

DNA Life (2018) Who we are. Retrieved from:

http://www.dnalife.healthcare/about-us/

Kashi Labs (n.d.)Weight management. Retrieved from:

https://kashilab.com/weight-management

Reasoner, J. (2015) Leaky gut syndrome in plain English – And how to fix it. Retrieved from: http://scdlifestyle.com/2010/03/the-scd-diet-and-leaky-gut-syndrome.

Swanson, N, Leu, A., Abrahamson, J, et. al. (2014) genetically engineered crops, glyphosate and the deterioration of health in the United States of America.Journal of Organic Systems. Retrieved from:

http://www.organic-systems.org/journal/92/abstracts/Swanson-et-al.html.9(2).

STEP 4: ENVIRONMENT

Clean 15. (n.d.). Retrieved from:

https://www.ewg.org/foodnews/clean-fifteen.php
https://www.ewg.org/foodnews/dirty-dozen.php

Dirty Dozen. (n.d.). Retrieved from:

https://www.ewg.org/foodnews/dirty-dozen.php

Filidei, M. (2000-2018). Toxic metals and mental health. A Guide to Alternative Mental Health. Retrieved from:

https://www.alternativementalhealth.com/toxic-metals-and-mental-health/

Martino, J. (2017). 15 foods that contain the mother of all antioxidants. Real Farmacy. Retrieved from:

http://realfarmacy.com/this-is-the-mother-of-all-antioxidants/

Story, C.M. (2014). Lead, mercury, arsenic in your body—10 tips to flush the toxins out. Renegade Health. Retrieved from:

http://renegadehealth.com/blog/2014/11/24/lead-mercury-arsenic-in-your-body-10-tips-to-flush-the-toxins-out

Web MD (2005-2018). Retrieved from:

https://www.webmd.com/diet/supplement-guide-alpha-lipoic-acid#1

STEP 5: BALANCE YOUR HORMONES

Hansen, F. (2017). How do cortisol levels change throughout the day. The Adrenal Fatigue Solution. Retrieved from:

https://adrenalfatiguesolution.com/cortisol-levels-change-throughout-day/

STEP 6: EMOTIONAL HEALING

Aliff, A. (2012). 30 traits of an empath. The Awakened State. Retrieved from:

http://theawakenedstate.tumblr.com/post/33146742903/30-traits-of-an-empath

Orloff, J. (2017). How to cut an unhealthy bond with someone. Psychology Today.

https://www.psychologytoday.com/us/blog/the-empaths-survival-guide/201707/how-cut-unhealthy-bond-someone

Made in the USA
Lexington, KY
17 November 2019

57204317R00105